Apathy or Action
Small Choice. Big Impact!

Exactly five months ago, I got the call. The call I'd been anxiously waiting for since I'd felt the small lump on my neck. I was at work, so I quickly walked into a quiet room. My heart was pounding out of my chest.

"Damon, you've got cancer."

Immediately, I was overwhelmed with fear and the tears started flowing. What about my kids? What about my wife who'd survived cancer twice? What would they do when I was no longer alive? Who would walk my daughters down the aisle at their weddings? Who would teach my son how to be a man? Who would love and protect my family when I was gone?

I rushed home to tell my wife before the kids got home.

"Honey, I have cancer."

We held each other tightly, our tears bonding our souls together.

"We'll get through this, we'll get stronger, and God will be glorified," I said as I looked her in the eyes.

I didn't plan on writing a book during my cancer journey. It just happened. It turns out it was one of the best decisions of my life. Writing helped me process my own emotions and make decisions through my journey. More importantly, I received overwhelming feedback from my blog that my writing was very inspirational to many people.

When I started writing I had no idea how many chapters would be in the book. "I'll be done writing when the story is over," I told people. My treatment is over and I'm cancer free. My story of overcoming cancer is now complete.

I don't know what your story is, but my prayer is that my story will inspire you as well.

Damon Stoddard

10/28/2019

Apathy or Action

Small Choice. Big Impact!

Dedicated to my wife, Debbie Stoddard

Debbie,

I love you with all my heart. We've built the family of our dreams together. It hasn't been easy. I watched you battle cancer and win. You never complained and you never lost faith. You just did what had to be done and you beat it. When cancer came back, I once again watched you battle it, and you won. I watched you conquer your fear by lifting your eyes upward and praising Jesus in the storm. And I've watched you continue to serve our family and everyone around you through it all.

When I discovered that I had cancer, our son, Nathan's response sums it up. "Dad, I'm not worried. Mom beat it twice and you will too."

Thank you, Debbie, for your inspiration. Thank you for loving me and standing by me when I'm at my best and when I'm at my worst.

I love you and I'm looking forward to spending the next 40 or so years together before we are together for eternity!

Damon

Contents

CHAPTER 1

5/30/2019

I Will Praise You in the Storm

I lift my eyes up to the hills—where does my help come from? My help comes from the Lord, the Maker of heaven and earth.
— Psalm 121:1-2

"Dad, guess what my memory verse is this week?" Nathan asked, sitting at breakfast the morning of my PET Scan to determine the extent of the cancer we'd discovered just two days earlier.

After rattling off a few verses, I finally surrendered. "I don't know," I responded.

"Come on dad, you know. It's from the biggest book in the Bible."

That makes it easier, at least it's from the Psalms. I guessed a few verses.

Psalm 40:1-3: "I waited patiently for the LORD; He turned to me and heard my cry. He lifted me out of the slimy pit, out of the mud and mire; He set my feet on a rock and gave me a firm place to stand. He put a new song in my mouth, a hymn of praise to our God. Many will see and fear the LORD and put their trust in him."

"Nope, that's not it."

Psalm 1:3: "He will be like a tree planted by streams of water, which yields its fruit in its season and its leaf does not wither; and in whatever He does, He prospers."

"Nope, that's not it. Here's another clue. It's from a song by Casting Crowns."

"Ahh…I know, As Far as the East is from the West!"

Psalm 103:12: "He has removed our sins as far from us as the east is from the west."

"Nope, that's not it either."

"I know what it is!"

Psalm 121:1!

"That's it!" he said as I asked him to read it out loud.

Psalm 121: "I lift my eyes up to the hills—where does my help come from? My help comes from the Lord, the Maker of heaven and earth"

Tears welled up in my eyes. My son knows one of my favorite songs, and the Lord knew I needed this song and my son's encouragement today.

Lord, I'm choosing to lift my eyes up to the hills today. I'm choosing to raise my hands to You. I'm choosing to praise You in this storm.

This is a storm that I've never endured before, but a storm that I've watched those very close to me endure. Nearly a year ago, my wife underwent major surgery to remove cancer. The cancer that arrived without a notice six years prior. The same cancer that the oncologist said was the "most treatable form of cancer on the planet." The same cancer that was pronounced gone from her body only a few months later after chemo and radiation.

But it wasn't gone. It came back with a fury the second time. The doctor shared that he wasn't concerned as my wife entered the biopsy. About an hour later, he looked deeply troubled. I knew something wasn't right.

"It looks like it was cancer, and it has grown very fast since we discovered it. I think I cut it all out, but we'll know for certain after the biopsy. It's a good thing you came in so quickly this time."

It's a good thing you came in so early this time. These words rang in my head as I remembered my sister undergoing radiation therapy 40+ years earlier to treat cancer of her lymph nodes. She only had a 20% chance of surviving, but by God's grace, she is alive and cancer free today. I remember the doctors saying, "it's a good thing you came in early; she might not be here today if you hadn't."

At my wife's follow-up appointment a few days later, the doctor pronounced he had successfully removed all the cancer and there was none at the margins. We both sighed a big sigh of relief, knowing we'd just dodged another bullet. As a precaution, we scheduled our meeting with the oncologist, believing we were done, and this would be a brief meeting to pronounce everything clear.

After all, this was the most treatable form of cancer on the planet.

I have a saying that has served me well over the years. A saying that I teach almost everyone I meet. A saying that I learned as the quality manager for Xbox 360 before we lost $1.5 billion in warranty costs from the largest reliability issue in history.

Quality is the gap between expectation and experience. If your experience exceeds your expectation, you are delighted. If your experience is less than your expectation, you are frustrated.

I've modified this slightly as a description for human emotion.

Emotion=Expectation minus Experience

We entered the oncologist's office with an expectation that no more treatment would be necessary. We had the expectation that our lives would continue as normal and this second round of cancer was just another blip.

Our expectation didn't match our experience when we heard the doctor's recommendation. Our emotions immediately changed. Peace was immediately replaced with fear.

It's very rare, but somehow the squamous cancer returned. This wasn't a recurrence of the original cancer; this was a new instance of the same form of cancer. This time it came back and was growing fast.

"The good news is we can treat it. It's a good thing you came in early because if you had waited it might have spread to her lymph nodes and it wouldn't have been treatable."

Our jaws hit the floor. We'd narrowly escaped another bullet.

The oncologist pulled out the recommended treatment. He shared the flow chart, the statistics, and his finger traced to the part that said surgery. Major surgery, the type of surgery that would require me to take a month off work to care for Debbie in her recovery.

Emotion=Expectation minus Experience

A year later, Debbie was pronounced cancer free. The surgery and treatment worked, again.

A few days after she was pronounced cancer free, I was rubbing my neck. Something felt suspicious. I felt a small lump, a little larger than a peanut just over my right carotid vein.

Immediately, I was gripped with fear. I tried to schedule a doctor's appointment the same day. Nothing available. I put it off for a few days but ultimately those words I'd heard so many times before rang in my ears.

"It's a good thing you came in early."

My wife is by my side because we went in early. My sister is 40+ years cancer free because my mom brought her in early.

I called and saw the doctor that afternoon.

"I'm not concerned. Give me a call in a week if it doesn't change size."

I decided to schedule an appointment in a week instead and get my annual checkup.

"It hasn't changed size, but I'm still not concerned. I'm going to schedule a CT scan to make sure. It's more for you than me."

A little more than 24 hours later, laying on the table as the CT machine scanned my neck, I had those same thoughts.

"Don't mess around Damon. It's good that you came in early."

"We'll get the results to your doctor and he will contact you."

The waiting is the hardest part.

I remember when my wife, Debbie, asked me to come upstairs. It was September 8, 2013. Just two days after one of the best days of my life, the day when I rode my bike 100 miles for the first time ever, and just a few short months after I'd competed in my first triathlon. Life was really good. My daughter, Monica, was back home, and after years of struggling with drug addiction, she was finally on her way to becoming healthy. Debbie was homeschooling our younger children, Nathan and Noelle, and our oldest daughter, Amanda, was working her way through college.

Life was better than it had ever been…

"Honey, I have cancer."

Her words pierced my soul and we laid on our bed holding each other, sobbing uncontrollably. Thoughts raced through my head. How would I raise our children alone? How would our children respond? How could we protect them from the emotional anguish associated with cancer?

In an instant our souls were knitted together, and I felt like she and I were one. We cried out to God begging him to save her.

The waiting is the hardest part.

For two weeks we anguished, cried, prayed, and held each other, waiting for the appointment with the oncologist. Those two weeks felt like 10 years.

The news was better than anything we'd hoped for. Her cancer was only stage one, and it was the "most treatable form of cancer on the planet." A little radiation, a little chemo, and she'd be good as new.

And just like that, a few months later she was pronounced cancer free.

As I write this, I'm having a Déjà vu.

The waiting is the hardest part.

The doctor contacted me a week after the CT scan. "I don't see anything but I'm going to refer you to a specialist."

Fortunately, this wait was only a few hours. The ear, nose, and throat specialist was available. I scheduled the appointment. She came in and immediately I felt peace.

"Damon, it doesn't look like cancer; but because of your history, I want to make sure. I'm going to schedule a needle biopsy under ultrasound to make certain there are no false negative readings."

The soonest appointment was the following Tuesday.

Seven more days of waiting.

The waiting is the hardest part.

Lying on the table, the doctor numbed my neck and pushed a needle in to collect a few samples. After it was over, he commented, "Man, you have tough skin. I really had to push the needle hard to get a sample!"

You should get the results within two to five business days.

More waiting.

I held my phone constantly, waiting for the call. And then it came. I was in a meeting at work, so I left the meeting to take the call. I answered and walked into a quiet conference room. My heart started beating so hard that I felt it would bounce out of my chest.

"Damon, are you somewhere where you can be alone?"

My heart started beating faster, I knew what she was going to say. Here we go again…

"Damon, you've got cancer."

As I type this, I'm waiting for my PET scan to determine the extent of my cancer.

The waiting is the hardest part.

Lord Jesus, I know You hold my life in the palm of Your hands. Lord, I've watched You work miracle after miracle after miracle in my life. Lord, thank You for my son's memory verse today. Today I choose to lift my eyes up to the hills. I know where my help comes from, it comes from You, Lord. The maker of heaven and earth. Lord, You have brought me and my family through many storms. This is another.

> And I'll praise You in this storm
> And I will lift my hands
> That You are who You are
> No matter where I am
> And every tear I've cried
> You hold in Your hand
> You never left my side
> And though my heart is torn
> I will praise You in this storm[i]

Questions to Consider

1. What is the storm you are facing in your life?

2. What is your greatest fear as it relates to this storm?

3. What choices can you make in the middle of the storm that will carry you through the storm?

4. What are you thankful for today?

5. How can I help?

CHAPTER 2

5/31/2019

The Peace of God that Transcends All Understanding

Be anxious for nothing, but in everything by prayer and supplication, with thanksgiving, let your requests be made known to God. And the peace of God, which surpasses all comprehension, will guard your hearts and your minds in Christ Jesus.
— Philippians 4:6-7

In my first book, *Pain Drives Change*[ii], I shared how God used the pain of separation, and ultimately divorce, to change me from the inside out into the man I am today. I talk briefly about the men in my life who carried me in a season when I felt all alone. I will be forever grateful to Bob and Steve for serving me with a selfless love and teaching me how to be a man of God.

That was 20 years ago. Bob and Steve were the only men in my life. But Bob introduced me to some great men. Through these men I met other great men and before I knew it, I looked around and realized I was surrounded by dozens of incredible men. Men who would (and have) dropped everything to support and encourage me.

It's been less than 72 hours since I was diagnosed with cancer and already I'm overwhelmed with the love and support I've received from these men.

Bob called me back almost immediately. I could hear the pain in his voice when I whimpered out those words, "I have cancer." He asked if I wanted to have lunch, much like he did 20 years ago when I shared that I was separated from my wife. He reminded me that his phone was on 24 hours a day and I could call if I needed anything. I know from experience these were more than words; he genuinely meant it.

Scott dropped everything and listened as I almost inaudibly said, "I have cancer." I could feel his tears on the other end of the phone, and when he said he would do anything to support and encourage me, I knew he meant it. And I knew his prayers would be earnest and continuous.

Dave responded immediately as well. As a man of great faith, he reminded me that God is the great healer and that he had personally experienced healing in hundreds of people. I left the call feeling great hope in my future.

Chuck answered in disbelief, but then quickly went into fervent prayer with me on the phone. Soon after, his wife offered to take care of our children at any time if we should need it. I've received several texts from Chuck over the last few days, always reminding me that he is praying for me and has assembled an army with his mom to pray for me as well.

Don was fishing and out of cell range (fishing for Halibut in Alaska!) but when he saw my text, he immediately responded. He promised to pray for me, and I know he will. He prayed for healing over my wife during her second bout of cancer and I'm certain God interceded to free her of cancer through his prayers.

My boss, Sean, responded to my text when I told him I was going to be late for a meeting. He encouraged me to take the day off. His support continues to overwhelm me, reminding me that he and Microsoft will do everything possible to help me through this. I know he means it because he did everything possible, including giving me a month off to care for my wife last year during her recovery from cancer. He reminded me again today, "Whatever you need, you've got."

Greg answered and was overwhelmed with joy to hear from me. When I shared that I had cancer, his tone shifted to genuine love and concern. He immediately went into prayer with me on the phone and prayed a very powerful prayer for me, a prayer to save my life so I could continue to build my family and expand His kingdom. Greg encouraged me to take the day off and process everything, and I took his advice. I thanked him for his wisdom and guidance in my life (encouraging me to write my first book and become a coach).

Fred was overwhelmed with disbelief and grief. I could feel his love and compassion as we talked on the phone. Fred asked if he could assemble a group of people to lay hands on me and pray over me at church, a gesture that touched me deeply. He texted me later in the day and shared that he could barely focus on work, but that he was praying fervently on my behalf. When I arrived for my PET scan, he was sitting there waiting for me. He reminded me that I wasn't alone, hugged me, and grabbed my hand as he prayed over me openly in the lobby!

The men I coach in Change YOUniversity responded immediately in prayer and encouragement. My co-workers have offered to help in any way possible. One of them even said he'd bring me whatever food I wanted if I felt trapped at home!

Steve picked up the phone and was pleasantly surprised to hear from me. After a few minutes of catching up, I shared that I had cancer. Always the engineer, Steve quickly shared his grief, and then quickly jumped into engineer mode, reminding me that cancer is very treatable today and that the science of understanding cancer and how to treat it has improved dramatically. He reminded me of how big God is and that He can cure this cancer. He then did as Steve often does. He told me how proud he was of me and reminded me of how much it means to him that I'd call and share.

Steve said he couldn't do much, but he would pray. I remember Steve's prayers; they were always powerful, and after he prayed, there always seemed to be a breakthrough. He is the righteous man from the book of James, "The prayer of a righteous man availeth much." I invited Steve to join us on Sunday when many people would be laying hands on me. He responded in typical Steve fashion. "You never know. I might just be out for a drive and show up."

To say that I'm blessed with people who love me and care deeply for me and my family is an understatement. As of this writing I've only shared this news with a few people, and I'm overwhelmed with their love and support. I hope to blog openly through this journey, and I'm certain that when I share more broadly, I'll be reminded of how many people God has put in my path and blessed me with.

As I am writing this, I'm preparing to reach out to Joe. As my pastor, Joe prayed over me at the altar at Cedar Park Church as the Holy Spirit transformed me into the man I've become. It's been almost 20 years, but I can still hear Joe's words that he always closed services with, the same words that describe how I'm feeling as I write this.

"And may the peace of God that transcends all understanding guard your hearts and minds forevermore."

Joe answered the phone and shared how good it was to hear from me. He congratulated me on my recent coaching certificate and asked how I was doing. I thanked him for how he always closed services and told him those words from Philippians were bringing me enormous peace. I shared that I couldn't explain it, but I was experiencing the peace of God that transcends all understanding. Then he prayed. WOW! I'd forgotten how powerful Joe's prayers were, but as he prayed, I could feel the Holy Spirit surround me and bring me peace. He prayed that I would find rest in green fields. Interesting, I've found enormous peace sitting on my deck in front of the fire and looking at my "green field," my backyard.

I heard back from Boyd today. We had a great talk as we haven't chatted for a few months. When I shared that I have cancer, he was shocked. He's walked through many trials with me and he reminded me that the trials just keep coming at me. He also reminded me that my ability to find peace in the trials has always impressed him. Then he prayed and declared Isaiah 26:3: "You will keep in perfect peace those whose eyes are fixed on you."

• • •

I received the news Tuesday that I had cancer. I waited a week for the results of the biopsy and every day of the week before I heard the news, I felt my anxiety increasing. My anxiety continued increasing for a few minutes after I heard the news.

I have cancer. It's in my lymph node. Will I die?

What will my kids do without a dad? Will my wife be ok? How will my older children handle the news? How severe is the cancer? When will I know?

Uncertainty leads to Anxiety

As simple as it sounds, anxiety stems from uncertainty. In life, there are few things you'll face that produce more uncertainty than the news of cancer. The uncertainty about whether you will live or die and the impact on your family produces a level of anxiety that is difficult to explain.

I'm sure you are asking the question, "Why are you writing a chapter called the peace of God that transcends all understanding if just three days ago you were overwhelmed with fear?" That's a great question.

A question for which I don't have an easy answer.

Why do I have so much peace when I have cancer that could easily take my life?

I have so many questions with no obvious answers.

- Why did I feel the lump in my neck?
- Why did I push the doctor so hard when he was certain it wasn't cancer?

- Why did the specialist choose a needle biopsy when she wasn't concerned?

- Why did the needle biopsy find the tiny location where the cancer resided?

- Why did my resting heart rate increase by seven points in seven days to the highest it had been in a year in the days waiting for the results of the needle biopsy?

- Why did it plummet the same seven points after I received the news I was diagnosed with cancer?

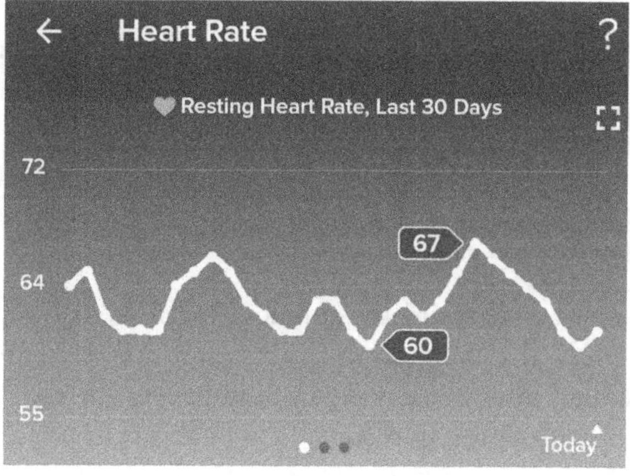

It's easy to SAY I'm experiencing the peace of God that transcends all understanding, but my resting heart rate is the data that supports my statement. I've been tracking my resting heart rate for about a year and a half and I've discovered that my sense of internal peace is DIRECTLY correlated with my resting heart rate. Even a single point increase or decrease in my resting heart rate predicts my overall anxiety, and even others can see the difference in my demeanor when my resting heart rate is low!

Uncertainty Leads to Anxiety but Predictability Brings Peace

It's undeniable. As I sit here writing this, I am 4.5 hours from my doctor's appointment. The results came in yesterday, the nurse's assistant called and said the doctor wanted to see me today, and she was making room in her schedule to do so. In 4.5 hours, I'll be sitting in her office and she will share the results of my PET Scan. The results could say that it hasn't spread, or the results could say that the cancer is terminal.

I don't know what they will say, but I know this…

God's got this! I've walked through trial after trial after trial in my life. Debbie and I have walked through trial after trial after trial in our lives. And we ALWAYS make it through. We lean into Him in our trials, we pray for His will to be done, we lift our hands up to the heavens, and we pray that He would be glorified through our trials. And He refines us. Our trials strengthen our faith as James 1:2-4 promises.

> *Consider it all joy, my brethren, when you encounter various trials, knowing that the testing of your faith produces endurance. And let endurance have its perfect result, so that you may be perfect and complete, lacking in nothing.*
> — James 1:2-4

And this trial is another refinement.

Predictability Brings Peace

I feel the peace of God that transcends all understanding as I sit here and write this. Predictability brings peace, yet NOTHING about my situation is predictable. But there is one thing that is predictable. God's got this. No matter what the prognosis is today, He will be glorified. The opposite of fear is faith. My faith in God in this trial gives me absolute predictability that He's in control of my life. He holds my life in His hands, and He will be glorified in this.

Thank you, Jesus, for the peace that transcends all understanding. Thank you, Jesus, that I know you and I know YOU've got this. Thank you, Jesus, that I'm not alone, that You've surrounded me with men who love me and are carrying me. Thank you for the text I just received from Fred. Thank you that I feel your arms tightly around me. Thank you for my band of brothers who are praying for me and my family, and thank you that I'm NOT alone.

8:19 AM

See this: As you walk today, Jesus is by your side with his arm tightly around you. Your helpmate is on other side doing same. Your band of brothers are all packed in very tightly around you, touching and holding you. We are all moving as a pack today. You are not alone my brother. You are NOT alone.

9:23 AM

Thank you Fred. I feel peace, the peace of God that transcends all understanding. I appreciate you.

Lord, as I sit in my office, I am listening to worship music and I feel close to you. I listen to the words and they penetrate my soul and draw me even closer to you. I am raising my hands to the heavens and I'm singing Hallelujah, You are my God.

In Your Presence[iii]

As I stand here in Your presence
Of Your beauty, I will always stand in awe
I reach my hands out to the heavens, yeah,
And I lift my voice to You alone.
To You alone
As I bow my head before You,
I lay my burdens down at Your nail pierced feet,
Every ounce of You
Radiates Your glory,
With You, I know that I am complete.
And I sing Hallelujah,
You are my God,
Maker of heavens,
Hallelujah, You are my Lord,
I bow before Your presence, yeah.
As I stand here in Your presence,
Of Your beauty I will always stand in awe,
I reach my hands out to the heavens, yeah,
And I lift my voice to You alone
And I sing Hallelujah,
You are my God,
Maker of the heavens,
Hallelujah
You are the Lord of all,
Maker of all the heavens,
I can only kneel before Your presence,
All the nations praise Your Holy Name
You are the great I Am,
More than I can reason,
I realize more that I am needing You
You are worthy, You are worthy
Lord

You are worthy, You are worthy,
You are mighty, You are mighty,
You are mighty, You are holy,
You are mighty, You are holy

For I know the plans I have for you, plans to prosper you and not harm you, plans for a future and a hope
— Jeremiah 29:11

Father, I rest in Your promise that You plan to prosper me and not harm me. I proclaim this promise and I hold it in my heart as I head out to have lunch with my wife before the prognosis.

I'm writing BEFORE my doctor's appointment when we will hear the results of my PET Scan. I'm writing it down as Habakkuk 2:2-3 says so that it WILL come to pass.

Then the Lord answered me and said, "Record the vision and inscribe it on tablets that the one who reads it may run. For the vision is yet for the appointed time; it hastens toward the goal and it will not fail. Though it tarries, wait for it; for it will certainly come, it will not delay."
— Habakkuk 2:2-3

Our lives are characterized by faith.

Faith in our family. Debbie and I lived by faith when our first marriages failed. We lived by faith when we realized Monica and Amanda would be raised without their biological mother and father being together. We lived by faith when Debbie feared that she couldn't have children with me, and we watched as He brought two beautiful children into our lives. We lived by faith when Monica struggled with drug addiction, and we watched in faith as He freed her from addiction and brought her home.

Faith in our health. We lived by faith when Debbie was diagnosed with cancer, and we watched as her body was healed. We lived by faith when I struggled with depression and overcame it. We lived in faith as Debbie was diagnosed with cancer a second time, and we watched in faith as her body was once again cured.

Faith in our finances. We lived by faith when I was laid off from Microsoft, and we watched in faith as He made a way for me to write my book in this time. We lived in faith that He would provide for us, and we watched in faith as He brought me back to Microsoft five months later with more money in the bank and a better job than I left. We lived in faith as we walked through a lawsuit for nearly five years, and we watched in faith as He grew our faith and ultimately enabled a settlement to be mediated outside of court.

Faith in our future. We lived in faith as I was diagnosed with cancer, and we walked in faith as he drew us closer. We watched Him cure my cancer and we experienced a deeper faith than we'd ever known. We lived by faith as He opened doors for ministry, and we walked in faith through those doors. We lived by faith as we raised our children to love Him and live for Him, and we grew our faith as they made it through their teenage years.

Our lives are characterized by faith. Faith as our fruit. We lived by faith as we watched the fruit that He bore through us. Fruit that came from our faith. Fruit in our children and through our children's lives. Fruit in our ministry. Fruit in the people's lives we touched and the hope that was restored because of our faith and our stories of how He carried us through our difficult times. Fruit in our grandchildren's lives as they experienced the joy of growing up in homes that were filled with love and free of dysfunction. Fruit in our great grandchildren's lives as they, too, experience the blessings of growing up in homes where faith was the bedrock and foundation.

In faith I proclaim that we will grow old together and enjoy the family we built. Debbie and I are sitting in our backyard. We are in our nineties. Our health is strong, our faith is stronger, and our family is whole. We watch our great grandchildren playing together in our yard under that same hundred-year-old shade tree I wrote about so many years ago. We are all together, our love for one another, and our love of Christ knits our hearts as one. Peace, love, joy. These embody my dream, the dream that I proclaim today on June 4, 2019, will come to pass!

Questions to Consider

1. Do you have a group of people in your life that surround you when the storms of life hit?
   If not, what action can you take to begin building this group?

2. Are you overwhelmed with fear from the storms in your life? How does your faith impact this fear?

3. How did your faith carry you through previous storms in life? How did these storms impact the person you are today?

4. What is your dream for your life? Is it written down? How often do you read it?

5. What are you thankful for today?

6. How can I help?

CHAPTER 3

06/27/2019

Butcher Knives and Hot Coals

Therefore, to keep me from becoming conceited, I am forced to deal with a recurring problem....
— 2 Corinthians 12:7

I love *Star Trek*. I watched it as a kid. I loved how Bones was always there with his handy dandy medical device. Just wave that wand over someone when they were injured and poof! Just like magic, the ailment was treated, and the patient was miraculously cured.

As an adult, I was so excited when they came out with *Star Trek*, the movie. You might remember *Star Trek IV - The Voyage Home*[iv]. The crew of the USS Enterprise needed to go back in time to save the whale. Chekhov had a brain injury and was lying unconscious in the operating room. Bones rushes up to the operating room to find the brain surgeon with a drill. You can hear the drill as the RPMs wind up, preparing to drill a hole in Chekhov's head to relieve the pressure. Bones looks at the surgeon and has a dialog that

I've never forgotten (here's a clip from my favorite scene https://www.youtube.com/watch?v=1i3gp_aN1cs)!

"My God man!

Drilling holes in his head is not the answer.

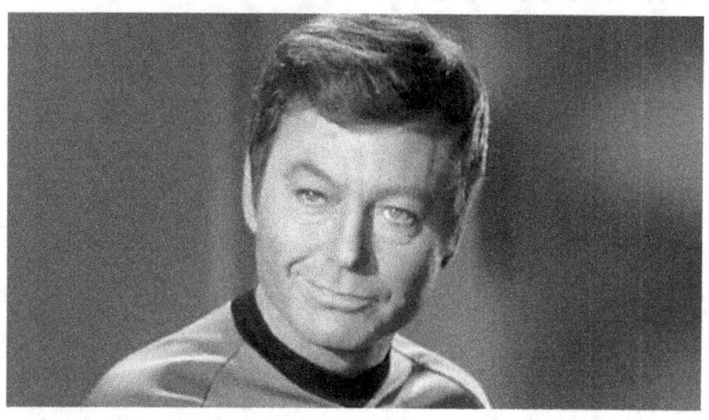

The artery must be repaired. Now put away your butcher knives and let me save this patient before it's too late! We're dealing with medievalism here! Chemo therapy...."

He then puts a gadget on Chekhov's head. Beep, beep, beep. Chekhov opens his eyes and he's healed!

Bones, I wish you were here a few years ago when my wife had to undergo chemotherapy and radiation for her first round of cancer treatment. I really wish you were here for the second round of medievalism when they pulled out the butcher knives and carved out the cancer.

me·di·e·val

[ˌmed(ē)ˈēvəl, ˌmēd(ē)ˈēvəl]

Definition: Very old-fashioned or primitive

I must admit, it does seem rather barbaric, old fashioned, and primitive. A small lymph node with a trace of cancer requires surgery? Debbie and I thought nothing of it—maybe a 30-minute procedure with a small incision.

Man, were we wrong. It's been eight days since the surgery and I finally feel decent enough to write this blog! Medication every four hours to stop the pain, unable to sleep more than two hours at a time, and talking hurts. Outside of a few short walks, I haven't exercised. All as a result of the surgery that left a six-inch scar wrapped halfway around my head!

Nathan and I have a running joke. Every time one of us gets a cut, we fist bump each other and say "man scar." This started when he was a toddler and smacked into a piece of rebar from sledding. It left a heck of a man scar on his face; he still has the scar today! Right before Debbie drove me to the hospital, I gave Nathan a fist bump and told him I was going to get a serious man scar. He smiled.

When the doctor came in, I joked with her saying, "I'd like a man scar please. Not a wimpy incision, but a real man scar."

She pulled her surgery pen out and sketched a line halfway around my neck.

I smiled and said, "Are you serious?"

She said she was serious. Surgery was going to be nearly three hours!

They wheeled me into the operating room. I smugly said, "I don't feel any anesthetic." A minute later (it was nearly three hours), I opened my eyes.

The next few hours were a blur, but I remember only wanting to see my wife. She stood by my bed giving me ice as I moaned from the pain in my throat where they'd removed my tonsils.

I love you Debbie Stoddard. You are always by my side, no matter what. You have cared for me selflessly and been strong when I struggled with the pain over the last few days. I don't know where I'd be without you. You are amazing. Thank you!!!!

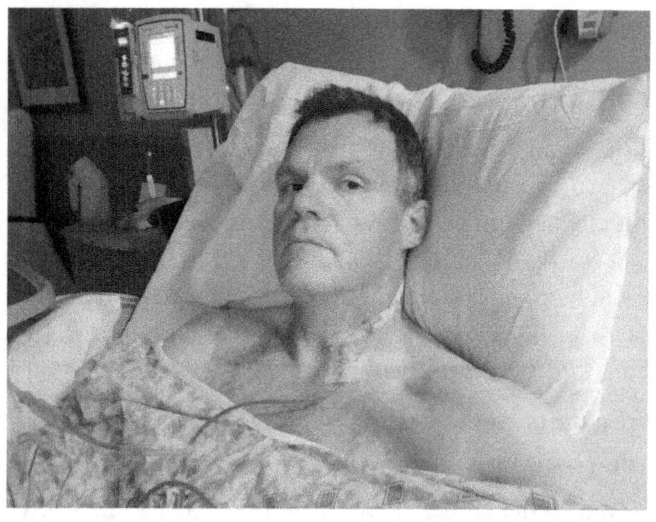

This picture above shows my "Man Scar" a few hours after surgery. The red tube is my bodily fluids being sucked out.

As Bones would say, "Cutting him open with a six-inch opening and removing a chunk of Stoddard steak isn't the answer."

Unfortunately, Bones would have been right. Yesterday, we finally received the pathology results. It turns out the "Stoddard steak" that was removed from my neck contained 18 lymph nodes. We knew one of the nodes was cancerous. They discovered another node was also cancerous, but the remaining nodes were cancer free. The cancer had started to spread, and the biopsy of the Stoddard steak revealed this. Fortunately (or unfortunately), the biopsy of my tonsils and the samples from my tongue didn't reveal any cancer.

"What does this mean?" I anxiously asked the doctor on the phone.

"It's good news, Damon. The prognosis for these situations is very good. Unfortunately, however, your treatment isn't over. We'll talk more about it on Thursday. For now, suffice it to say that you'll need radiation of your mouth and throat areas."

But what will they radiate? If there is no cancer, why radiate? "Medievalism," as Bones would say. Unfortunately, that's the state of our understanding of this type of cancer, and the only known cures are akin to medievalism! The butcher knives weren't enough to remove all the cancer, so now we resort to burning-hot coals! Radiation, that is. Radiation that literally fries all the tissue it touches, much like a medieval torture chamber with burning coals applied to the interior of my mouth and throat. A torture that I'm guessing will last for four to six weeks.

OK...enough sarcasm. In all honesty, it's true. Cancer treatment options are still very limited—butcher knives (surgery), poison (chemotherapy), and hot coals (radiation). But it's the best we have, and I thank God for the doctors that found this and their wisdom for the best-known treatment available to man today. Cut out a piece of Stoddard steak and fry all remaining tissue that could have been the source of the cancer in the lymph nodes.

My doctor tells me that cancer doesn't originate in the lymph nodes, it jumps there from somewhere else. Either the throat or the tongue or the tonsils. Since they were unable to detect it in my throat or tonsils or tongue, they are left with no options except to believe that it is so microscopic in the tissues that they can't detect it. To make sure it doesn't grow, they'll nuke the tissue and kill any cells that might have cancer. Unfortunately, they'll also kill some other cells. Namely, the cells that produce saliva and the cells that help me taste food.

Yesterday was a tough day to say the least. I didn't know whether I should rejoice or cry. Rejoice because cancer is removed or cry because I'm about to undergo some major radiation? Honestly, yesterday was perhaps the hardest day that I can remember in a very long time. Let me take a minute to explain why it was so hard to try and pull all this together.

It boils down to one simple word. Fear. Yes, the same fear that I talked about in my last blog, and so exuberantly stated I wasn't experiencing. But this time the fear is different than anything I've ever experienced. This time it wasn't the fear of loss or the fear of emotional pain. I've been through those and I wrote about my journey in my first book. My wife reminded me last night what this fear was about.

THE FEAR OF PHYSICAL PAIN

She reminded me that I've never really experienced much physical pain, so this is going to be a battle unlike any I've faced. Truth be known, I have faced a little bit of physical pain. It's been almost constant for the last eight days. Not severe (at its worst it was a six on a scale of one to ten). But it's been there for eight days.

Sometimes it goes away, and I feel normal. But I'm reminded of it when it's time to eat (I've lost five pounds this week because it's been so difficult to eat). I'm reminded of it when I talk. I'm reminded of it when I try to sleep. (I'm a back sleeper but am unable to sleep on my back right now because when I do, my throat doesn't have sufficient room for me to breathe and I begin to gag, feeling like I'm about to suffocate.) So, I sleep on my side, but every few hours I wake up (laying on my back), unable to breathe easily. I get up, drink my ice water, take some medicine, eliminate the water that has accumulated in my bladder, and lay back down on my side. A few hours later, the process begins again.

No, it hasn't been awful. It's been uncomfortable, and I've been excited that it was about to be over because I was healing. But then I got the call. As I processed it, I realized that what I've been going through the last eight days will start all over again in a few weeks. Except this time, it won't be over in eight days. It might be over in six to eight weeks. I don't know for sure; I'll find out tomorrow.

Yes, I'm experiencing fear of the impending physical pain. I held my son last night with tears in my eyes and I told him I feared the pain, but that I would be ok. I told him it was ok to have emotions as a boy, and I showed him through my own tears that I was experiencing deep emotions. *Lord, protect Nathan during this season. Let him learn lessons about You through his mom's and my battles with cancer that will grow his faith and help him be a man who fully trusts you.*

Yes, I'm experiencing fear of the impending physical pain. I held my daughter in my arms as she sobbed uncontrollably, afraid of her dad experiencing this pain. Worried that they wouldn't get all the cancer and that I might die. I reassured her that I wasn't going to die, but that I was choosing to focus on all the good versus the bad that could happen. In my fear, I comforted her and showed her how I am choosing to handle a situation that is completely out of my control. *Lord, protect Noelle during this season. Give her peace and comfort. Help her to learn from her mom and me how to relinquish control and trust You in the seasons of her life when things happen that are out of her control. Help her become a woman who fully trusts you.*

Yes, I'm experiencing fear of the impending physical pain. I won't be able to effectively coach my son's football team, and I likely won't be able to go salmon fishing with him and my father in law.

CANCER SUCKS!

However, my treatment and prognosis for a successful recovery are much better than the alternative.

A mentor reminded me of all the people who go through what I'm going through and don't have Jesus. WOW. Where would I be without my faith right now?

My wife reminded me of all the people that go through this and are all alone, without family. WOW. Where would I be without my family and friends right now?

My banker reminded me today of all the people who hear the news and have NOBODY to help. WOW.

Thank You, Jesus, for all the blessings You've bestowed upon me and my family.

Thank You that I have a family that loves me, that I have great medical insurance, that I have great doctors.

Thank You that my cancer was caught early, and that the Stoddard steak removed another lymph node with cancer.

Thank You that I have a wife who is caring for me and making sure that I am fed, and my medication is taken at the right time to minimize my pain. Thank You for her example of fully trusting and surrendering to You in her own battle with cancer, and how she's taught me to have faith in her own struggles with pain.

Thank You for my boss who texts me every couple of days and asks how I'm doing.

Thank You for my job that is paying for me to be off work and recover. Thank You for my medical benefits that are paying for the treatment.

Thank You for the men who laid hands on me and prayed before my surgery, and for the men who stopped by and said hi to me.

Thank You for my counselor and friend who stopped right before surgery and gave me a flower and prayed over me.

Thank You for my home and my backyard and gas firepit where I can sit and be warm and feel the peace of God that transcends all opportunity.

Thank You for the opportunity to write about this and the opportunity to inspire other people who might be struggling through the platform You've given me to reach many people.

Thank You in advance for the lives that will be saved because they randomly read my blog and were inspired to have that lump checked.

Thank You for my wife whose best friend is alive because my wife shared her cancer story, and for her cancer (the same that I have) being cured, and thank You for her encouraging texts to my wife for me as I undergo the same treatment she did.

Thank You that You, Jesus, endured more physical pain than I will ever endure, and because of it, the sins of my past are completely wiped clean and I have more peace and joy than I ever deserved.

And Jesus, thank You in advance for this new thorn in my side called cancer. Thank You that my faith is re-ignited whenever I'm in pain and see the opportunity to use my pain not only for my personal growth, but also for the growth of those who will one day endure the same hardship I am currently undergoing.

Thank You that my mom, so many years ago, taught me through her example to be thankful for everything through her daily journal writing. Thank You that she is in heaven with You and is no longer experiencing her pain.

When I heard the news yesterday, I had a choice to make. I could choose to focus on everything bad that will happen because of the radiation, or focus on everything good that will come from it. I allowed myself to focus on the fear for a short period of time. This fear paralyzed me.

Today, I choose faith. Even though Bones can't put the magic gadget on my neck and instantly cure this cancer,

I still choose faith. I choose to be thankful and focus on everything good, right, lovely and pure…and because of it the peace of God is with me!

> *Finally, brethren, whatever is true, whatever is honorable, whatever is right, whatever is pure, whatever is lovely, whatever is of good repute, if there is any excellence and if anything worthy of praise, dwell on these things.*
> — Philippians 4:8

Questions to Consider

1. What is your greatest fear?

2. How can you shift your focus from fear to everything you are thankful for?

3. How can I help?

CHAPTER 4

7/9/2019

The Good News and the Bad News

"Damon, you must have a guardian angel. It's a miracle that your cancer was caught so early. I wish all my patients were as proactive as you are."
— Nancy (My Nurse Navigator)

A few years ago, our church had a family camp in Wenatchee, Washington, over the Fourth of July. My good friend, Kyle, was going, so we decided to drag our trailer across the mountains and hang out in the baking sun in the middle of the fairgrounds! We had an awesome time that year and discovered a few things that we loved. There is an incredible bike trail (The Apple Loop Trail) that goes around the Columbia River, through the desert, across bridges, and into Walla Walla park along the Columbia River. AWESOME would be the understatement of the century. A 25-mile bike loop in the area where I grew up as a kid is soul food. We also discovered the best Fourth of July fireworks show in the park, with the Wenatchee Valley Orchestra playing live.

Like many areas of my life, I knew I needed to build a routine around going to Wenatchee every Fourth of July. A "system" of rest and relaxation to fill my soul and bond with my family. The timing this year couldn't have been better.

I was able to start riding my bike again a few days earlier, and my body and emotions needed to recover from the trauma associated with my surgery. Furthermore, I needed to process the news from a few weeks later that my treatment wasn't over; it had, in fact, just begun.

As I write this, I've just returned from a four night camping trip in Wenatchee. I feel rested and at peace. People at work asked me how I'm doing. "100%," I say. Truth is, I feel 110% right now. One-hundred-ten percent, even though I'm entering a season that promises to be painful. One-hundred-ten percent because I proactively built a "system" into my life to recharge. Three long bike rides last week, with a brief stop to spill my emotions out to God, and experience that fear that creeps in when I allow myself to think of everything bad that will happen.

- What if this is my last bike ride here?
- What if the radiation leaves me with insufficient saliva to ride my bike?
- What if my neck is so stiff from the radiation that I can't bend it during my bike ride?
- What if…

I apologize for being crude, but years ago a good friend and mentor confronted me when I was stuck in the "what if" loop. He looked me right in the eye when I was looking at all the potential negative outcomes. What if…, What if…, What if…?

"Damon, what if monkeys fly out of my butt?" Yeah, it's possible. Anything is possible.

Point taken, Jeff. Thank you for the wakeup call so many years ago.

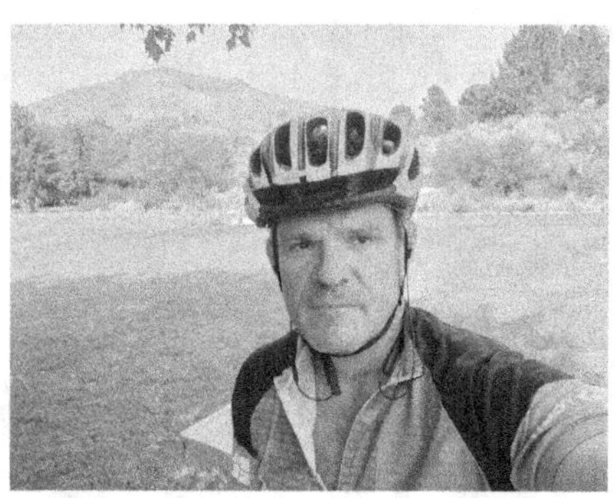

My tears flowed for a few brief minutes and I flushed out the "what ifs" from inside. Something about a good cry creates freedom. I jumped on my bike, and for the rest of the weekend, enjoyed my family. Boating and swimming in the ice cold water, ice cream, burgers, Cheeseburger Subs (dang, these are addicting!), boating on Lake Chelan, biking to fireworks with my kids, kayaking in the river, s'mores over the fire at night, and just hanging out with the people I love the most.

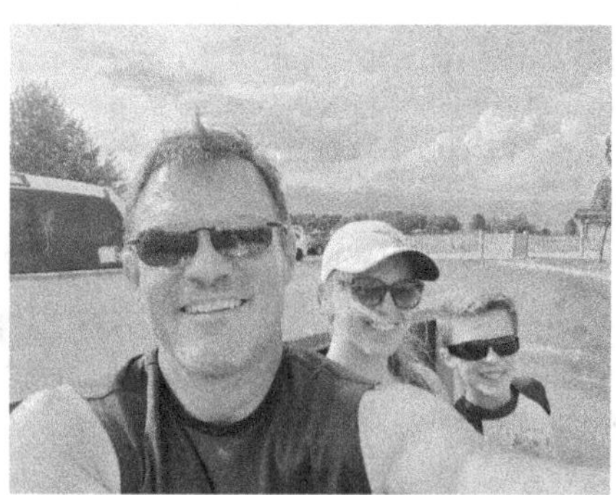

Thank You, Jesus, that years ago I discovered the power of systems and began implementing them in my life. Thank You for the system of family vacations in areas we love. The system that came at exactly the right time to rejuvenate me in preparation for the impending radiation treatment.

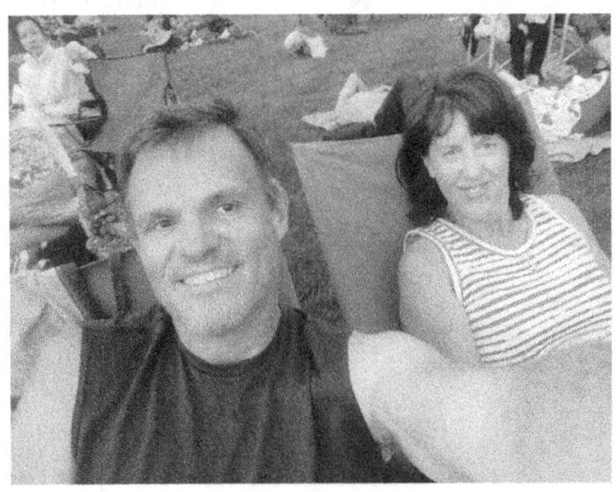

I'll talk a bit more about systems later as I've realized over the past few days how critical my personal "systems" are to my long-term health and vitality, particularly after radiation.

Let's rewind a few days and talk about the news I received as I was driving across the mountains on my way to the camping trip.

My phone rang just outside of Goldbar. I knew the number and was expecting the call, so I quickly answered it hoping that I wouldn't lose cell signal.

"Damon, it's Nancy, your nurse navigator. Is now a good time to talk?"

Immediately my heart started racing. I'd been expecting the call as the "cancer board" had met earlier in the day to discuss my case. I was waiting to hear if I needed chemotherapy in addition to my radiation.

"Damon, I've got some really good news and I've got some not-so-good news," Nancy said.

Just a few days earlier, I learned most of the details about my cancer and treatment from the radiation oncologist, but not all. Nancy was calling me to share the results of the cancer board discussion.

Before I share the news from Nancy's phone call, it's important to go back to the meeting with the radiation oncologist. For nearly two hours, my wife and I sat in a very comfortable room talking about my cancer, the treatment, and the side effects.

I entered the room thinking that I'd lose my taste buds forever and lose all saliva production forever. I was confident in overcoming cancer, but concerned about the side effects. I left the room elated to hear that food would only taste like cardboard for a few months after treatment. If everything worked out, I'd be able to taste the rolls and turkey on Thanksgiving.

And I was elated to hear that my saliva production would only go down by 30%. Unfortunately, this would be a long-term effect of radiation.

Now the details. The cancer I have is known as Squamous Cell Carcinoma. I'm going to share some details of what she shared as best as I can remember, but please don't interpret what I say below as fact. It is simply my recollection of what she shared.

Squamous Cell Carcinoma can be traced to HPV. That's Human Papillomavirus Infection. Yes, the type that is transmitted through sexual activity and so much more. Today, HPV is considered an epidemic as 90 to 95% of adults are carrying HPV and most don't even know it! The incidence of Squamous Cell Carcinoma is on the rise, yet it isn't understood why. All that is known is that HPV sometimes, in some people, mutates into cancer—Squamous Cell Cancer. Many times, it's 20 to 30 years after the unknown onset of HPV. How did I get it? Nobody knows.

The radiologist proceeded to share that there are a few different strains of this carcinoma: the positive strain and the negative strain. The negative strain is difficult to treat and has around a 40% survival rate. The positive strain, however, is very treatable and has a 90%+ success rate.

Guess which one I have? The positive strain. WAHOO!!!! This cancer is the kind that is treatable! I'm elated to hear this news, but quickly reminded of the same conversation in the same room six years earlier. My wife also had Squamous Cell Carcinoma, and the Oncologist stated that "it was the most treatable form of cancer on the planet." After she was treated with chemo and radiation, she was pronounced cancer free and we celebrated. Five years later, it returned as a new instance of the same cancer that was "the most treatable form of cancer on the planet." By the grace of God, she's been pronounced cancer free again, but she reminds me often that she is always wondering if it will come back again.

My cancer is very treatable. That's the good news. The bad news is that they were unable to find the source of the cancer. My cancer appeared in my lymph node, but this type of cancer doesn't start in the lymph node. It starts somewhere in the head and neck region. Most of the time, they can identify the source of the cancer and treat it directly.

Most of the time. The source of my cancer was not discovered, which only happens five to 10% of the time. So, the data for treatment of a cancer where the source is unknown is sparse.

"We're going to treat it with radiation. A general dose of radiation in your head and neck area every day for six weeks. Fortunately, because you caught it so early, we don't have to have a high dose of radiation. We can use a lower dose. But if all goes well, you'll be cancer free and the long-term outcome is very, very good."

"How painful will it be?" I asked.

"Your wife's cancer treatment was the most painful. Yours is right next to it as the most painful form of cancer treatment because of the location in your tongue and throat. The next three months are going to be challenging for you."

I smiled. "Bring it on."

It's very treatable. We caught it early, and there are only a few side effects: 30% saliva loss, short-term taste bud loss, stiffening of my neck, and potentially turkey neck.

Finally, she reminded me that I'd want to see a dentist quickly. My bones will be degraded in my head and neck. A tooth extraction after radiation could result in bone rot because it might never heal. (I wasn't concerned about this one because I haven't had a cavity in years.)

"Damon, I want to bring your case to the cancer board on Wednesday. I want to get everyone's opinion to make sure that your treatment plan is vetted with everyone. The recommended procedure is either do nothing or radiate. Because we don't know the source, my recommendation will be to radiate and potentially chemo. We'll talk on Wednesday and let you know!"

"I can do this," I told my wife as we walked out high fiving each other at the great news, excited but anxious about the outcome of the cancer review board on Wednesday.

Wednesday arrived and I got the call I was talking about earlier from Nancy.

"Did they review my case?"

"Oh yeah, they reviewed your case. They spent a lot of time talking about you. The best cancer doctors were there, and they talked and talked and talked and reached a consensus about your treatment."

"And?"

"You were proactive and caught this very early. This is great news. You caught it so early that nobody knows the original source of the cancer. Recall cancer doesn't start in the lymph nodes, it starts somewhere in your head and neck area. Our most senior doctors—he'll be your primary oncologist long term—was emphatic that the cancer originated in your tongue and it was simply too early to detect it. All of the oncologists believed that radiating the nasal passages would cause more harm than good, so you won't have to have this treatment. Furthermore, chemotherapy will not be necessary!"

"Wait, let me make sure I understand what you are saying. I won't need chemotherapy. This is great news. And did I hear you say that I won't need radiation?"

"No, that's not exactly true. You won't need radiation of the nasal passages, but you will need radiation in your tongue and throat."

"Ahh, got it. This is great news," I responded, even though I didn't know it was a possibility that I might need radiation in the nasal area.

"How did you find this, Damon?"

I described the series of events, starting with finding the lump, doctors not seeming worried, but eventually getting a biopsy that showed cancer.

"Wow. Thanks for sharing that story Damon. Now that I have the entire history, I want to remind you of how fortunate you are. This cancer is treatable, and because you caught it so early, it will be eliminated from your body. I'm not sure if you realized it, but the cancer is so early that you are fortunate that the biopsy caught it. There are a lot of cases where cancer is present and a biopsy doesn't catch it.

"Damon, you must have a guardian angel. It's a miracle that your cancer was caught so early. I wish all my patients were as proactive as you are," Nancy said.

We finished the call by setting a follow-up appointment with the medical oncologist. Furthermore, I shared with her that my friend Ted, who has undergone three rounds of cancer treatment, recommended that I be proactive and get a feeding tube implanted so that if I can't eat, my body will still have nourishment and we won't be reacting to get it nourishment. She agreed and promised to become my "advocate" behind the scenes to make this happen.

Lord, thank You for watching over me. Thank You that I felt the lump early. Thank You that I pushed through the argument in my head to not take the time off work and get it checked. Thank You that I didn't listen to the primary care physician and became my own advocate to know about my lump. Thank

You that he followed through, realized I needed a specialist, and sent me to her. Thank You that my sister went before me and her cancer inspired me to always have lumps checked. Thank You that the resultant biopsy came back positive when it could have easily been a false negative. Thank You that I was able to have the surgery and today I'm 110% recovered after only three weeks. Thank You that the radiologist spent the time with me and my wife, and that the doses can be moderate because it was so early. Thank You that I had the blessing of having my case thoroughly reviewed with the cancer board and there were many experts in that room. Thank You for my "Ted Talks," where I can learn and be inspired by a friend and man of great faith who

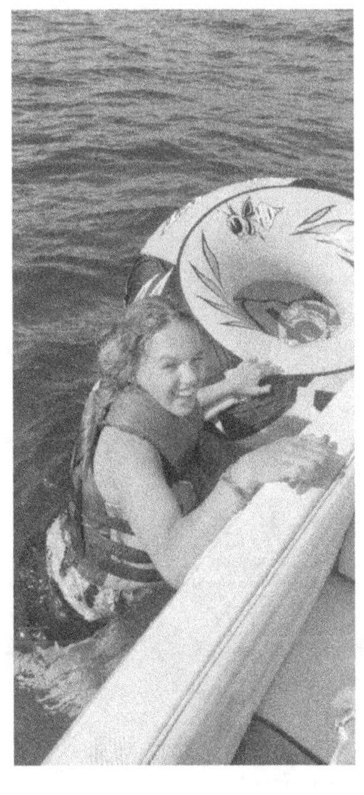

has walked this road multiple times before. Thank You for his example of faith amid his own cancer treatment and how it is inspiring my faith and desire to inspire others through my writing and example. Thank You for the rest I received over the weekend. Thank You for my job, my boss, my benefits, my health, my family, my friends, my faith, my church, and the gift of eternal optimism and positivity amid this storm. Thank You in advance that this cancer will be eradicated from my body for eternity and that I will have a story that will bring You glory.

Just one more major hurdle before getting the treatment started! My dentist appointment to learn the long-term impact on my oral health from the radiation.

Questions to Consider

1. What are the "what-ifs" you are experiencing?

2. What activities "feed your soul?" When was the last time you fed your soul?

3. How can I help?

CHAPTER 5

7/15/2019

Cancer of Unknown Primary Source (CUPS)

My wife reminded me that I haven't always had the best oral hygiene. When we were first married, I didn't brush my teeth in the evening because I was too lazy and too tired and clearly didn't know the impact of not brushing. Somewhere along the way, I discovered how important brushing is and started brushing in the evening as well as morning. It seems like it worked. No cavities in decades!

At least I thought it worked. My primary dentist retired about a year ago and I haven't bothered going back in for my twice-a-year checkup. However, when my radiation oncologist told me how critical it was to see the dentist, I took her advice and scheduled the appointment.

My new dentist introduced herself. She'd been practicing for a few years since graduating. I looked around the office and noticed all the equipment was new. When we took X-rays, they still placed the old-fashioned lead jacket on my chest, but this time the images showed up immediately on the large computer screen in the exam room. I hadn't really thought about it, but realized how much more effective digital images are. I also realized how much radiation I've already been exposed to with multiple CT scans of my head and neck region, and now the dental X-rays.

Cool technology, and great news! I didn't have any cavities. When my new dentist asked how frequently I floss, I let her know that I didn't floss.

"It shows. You have the early stages of gum disease."

Once again, the fear creeped in. Not because of gum disease. (Arguably, my own fault for not flossing regularly. My system is perfectly designed to give me gum disease.) No, the fear creeped in because she reminded me of the dangers of radiation.

Radiation weakens the bone structure in the jaw, and it's known as Osteoradionecrosis, or bone death due to radiation. The threat of Osteoradionecrosis, or ORN for short, put a deep fear in me. ORN reveals itself after a tooth needs to be extracted after you've had a certain dose of radiation. The problem is, once the tooth is extracted, there is a possibility that the wound will never heal, and it can begin rotting the bone. In some cases, parts of the jawbone need to be surgically removed.

My new dentist reminded me of ORN and reminded me that I needed to improve my oral hygiene immediately. Furthermore, I needed to start brushing with prescription toothpaste 30 minutes after each meal.

A text message with my sister confirmed my fears. Her radiation from 40 years ago resulted in a lot of dental problems.

Your system is perfectly designed to get you the results you are getting

My oral hygiene system of brushing twice a day and not flossing resulted in the start of gum disease. Further neglect of my oral hygiene after radiation treatment would be the perfect system to give me the potential of major problems in the future.

I've always struggled with flossing. Not anymore. I purchased eight toothbrushes and have ordered multiple containers of floss. The toothbrushes are strategically placed so that I always have one at hand after eating. The floss is also strategically placed. Furthermore, I've added three daily questions to my "morning habits" checksheet to ask if I've flossed and brushed the previous day. In the week since seeing the dentist, I've discovered that my "habit of daily habits" has made it very easy to add a new habit of flossing and brushing after each meal.

My new system is perfectly designed to protect my oral hygiene and should minimize the potential of ORN-induced infection. I fully understand the "why" of this change and I'm committed to this new habit for the rest of my life.

But wait…there's more!

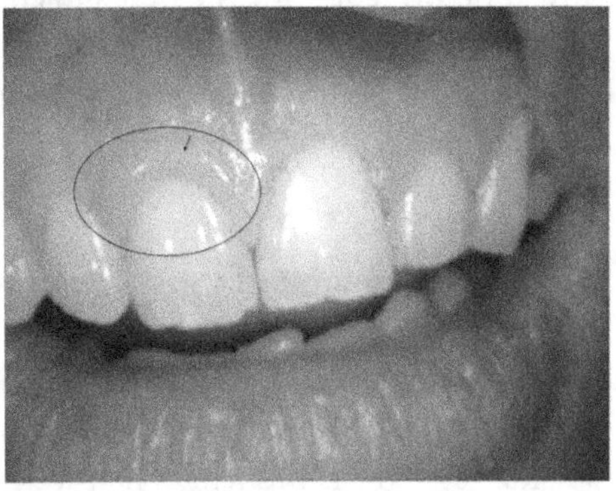

Apologies for the crude picture of my teeth, but I think it makes the point I'm about to make.

"Damon, you have a spot on your gums, and I'm concerned about it. I'm not an expert, but I want to make sure it isn't cancer."

Whack. Another slap to the face. Immediately, my mind started asking questions. Could this be the source of the cancer in my lymph nodes? The cancer they were unable to locate from the surgery and removal of the Stoddard steak, as well as the extraction of my tonsils? If yes, why didn't they tell me earlier? My mind was racing. I didn't know whether to be elated or deflated.

I called my wife and together we processed ORN, gum disease, and the potential that this new spot on my gums might be cancer. I love you Debbie Stoddard, I can't imagine walking this journey alone. I'm so blessed to have you as my wife, my life partner, as we walk through life "in sickness and health".

That was Monday night. By Tuesday morning I'd processed this new information. I implemented the new habits of brushing and flossing onto my daily habits' checklist. I scheduled my appointment with the oral surgeon for Friday, and I called my nurse navigator. She recommended a follow-up appointment with my ear, nose, and throat specialist, and I scheduled that for Thursday.

• • •

Forgive me for the tangent, but if you've been reading my blogs and/or my previous book, you'll notice a pattern. Pain drives change. The only question is how do we respond to change: I've learned in my life that pain is a signal that something in your life "system" is broken. When we experience this pain we have a choice: dwell on the pain and let fear engulf us, or accept the pain and allow God to make the changes in that need to be made.

I've learned to accept the pain and respond with action. Action is the best and strongest antidote for fear. Once again, I chose action, and because of the action, my potential suffering from pain is eliminated.

Truth be known, Tuesday—less than 12 hours after my dentist appointment—I felt more energized and optimistic than I had in a long time. By accepting the "pain," I eliminated the suffering.

Suffering=Pain-Acceptance

My friend taught me this a few months ago and it is very profound. When in pain, you can easily avoid suffering by simply accepting the situation. Furthermore, you can avoid the despair associated with suffering if you can apply meaning to your suffering.

Despair=Suffering-Meaning

I have decided to face this cancer battle by applying meaning to the brief bouts of suffering I experience from my pain.

The meaning I am gleaning from my cancer is crystal clear. I want to use my experience with cancer to provide hope and encouragement to people who are experiencing cancer, to reach people before cancer spreads, and to inspire them to get it checked. My writing has proven to be an incredible source of meaning for me, and the feedback I've already received from those who read about it has reinforced how meaningful my journey through cancer is to them.

A friend reached out to me recently. He'd started reading my book and was reading my blogs. As we sat and talked, he shared with me how meaningful my writing was to him. He shared that he had faced difficult situations in the past and responded differently than I am. He shared that he no longer wanted to be that way, and my writing was giving him a vision for his future. *Thank You, Jesus, for providing meaning to my journey through cancer. I pray You would make my journey and story available to anyone that it will help.*

Pain drives change.

Don't waste your pain by suffering.

Accept it.

Don't waste your pain by having no meaning. Use your pain to serve others. I guarantee your perspective will shift dramatically when you take action based on the meaning behind your pain.

OK. Sorry about that sidebar, I just thought it was important to share.

• • •

I arrived at my ENT's office Thursday morning. Her office was able to create an opening less than 12 hours after I'd requested it. We talked about the spot on my gums. She quickly looked and said she wasn't concerned. We talked about ORN. She reminded me that it was a very low likelihood. We talked about saliva loss and the surgery. She looked at me and said, "You'll be fine."

I left her office relieved and thankful for her expertise in identifying the cancer in my lymph node through the biopsy. I was relieved for a short period of time.

I decided to follow through with the appointment with the oral surgeon the next day. I entered his office and once again was incredibly impressed with his knowledge and compassion. He gave me a fist bump and a thorough oral exam. He confirmed my ENT's diagnosis. No cancer on my gums.

I asked him about ORN. He confirmed it can be bad, but said it is a function of the dosage of radiation, and said he'd have to know in order to give me the likelihood of occurrence. He ended the session by offering do it for free. I thanked him and reminded him that I have great insurance, so charging wasn't a problem.

After leaving the office I called my wife and we processed the news. The spot on my gums was not cancer, leaving us where we started a week ago. We didn't know the source of the cancer. Truth be known, we didn't even know if I still had cancer. There was a likelihood that the removal of my tonsils also removed the cancer, but they couldn't find the cancer because it was so early.

As we talked, the truth of it all began to set in and I once again started crying. I have cancer, or I at least have a high likelihood of cancer. The experts don't know exactly where to treat it, but they have a strong belief that my cancer originated in the base of my tongue. So, they've devised a treatment plan to maximize the likelihood of eliminating the cancer of unknown primary source. A treatment plan of six weeks of radiation with potential side effects of ORN, saliva loss, turkey neck, and six weeks of pain that would easily exceed what I'd previously experienced. A treatment plan that should have a high cure rate, but can't be known for certain because we still don't know the source.

I decided it was time to do some research. I've avoided research up until now because I didn't want to put survival rate numbers in my head that I couldn't remove. I couldn't avoid it any longer; I needed to do the research and understand this type of cancer a little deeper. I needed to understand why it wasn't located and determine if there were any other known treatment options. I needed to apply the 30 years of professional problem solving and statistical data analysis to my own problem, the problem known as CUPS (Cancer of Unknown Primary Source). And I needed to do it quickly. Monday would be the day when we finalized my treatment plan with the radiation oncologist. My wife agreed, and I got to work.

That was Friday. I'm writing this on Monday afternoon after my discussion with the radiation oncologist where we collectively decided to put my radiation treatment on pause and seek an emergency referral with UW Cancer Research. CUPS is very rare (between 1% and 10% of these types of cancers). Because of the rarity, my initial research indicated it would be prudent to seek another opinion.

I'll talk more about my research findings and my path forward next. Now it's time to sign-off. I have a date with my beautiful wife and I'm not going to be late!

Thank You, Jesus, for guiding my path in this cancer treatment. Thank You for the meaning You've helped me see and thank You for the people who are benefitting from sharing my story. Thank You for the peace I am experiencing and thank You that I have a little time to continue researching and get other opinions. Thank You for the people in my life who have encouraged me to seek out different opinions and thank You for the events leading up to my conviction to do so. Thank You for the quality of care I've received up until now and thank You for helping me find this cancer early. Thank You for the opportunity to write. Thank You for the opportunity to apply 30 years of professional problem-solving experience to my own cancer. Thank You for my curious and inquisitive nature and the ability to ask probing questions that many times lead to deeper understanding (even though they drive others crazy at times!). Thank You for the hope I'm feeling now as I wait for the referral appointment with the UW.

As my mom always used to write in her journal, "Guide me and protect me and my family on this journey."

Questions to Consider

1. Do you believe the statement, "Pain drives change?" How does it apply to your current situation?

2. Are you suffering? What do you need to do to accept the pain, thereby eliminating the suffering?

3. Are you feeling despair? What do you need to do to find meaning?

4. What action do you need to take to help you right now?

5. How can I help?

CHAPTER 6

7/17/2019

Carpe Data!

The last few days have been a whirlwind. On Monday, after talking with my radiation oncologist, we decided to pause on the creation of my face mask for radiation and seek out an opinion from the University of Washington about an alternate treatment approach that I discovered while doing some research. Yesterday, I met with my medical oncologist, and we confirmed that this alternate path was prudent with both oncologists saying, "If I were in your situation, I'd do exactly what you are doing. You have to have confidence in your treatment plan. Your life is dependent on these decisions, so do whatever you need to do to gain the confidence you need to proceed."

How did we arrive at this decision? We arrived because I decided to start researching and I brought the research to the experts. This research opened conversations and might have enlightened my oncologists with information they weren't intimate with.

I've spent my career solving big problems. I've been trained as an expert in a methodology known as Six Sigma, and

I've been certified as a Master Black Belt in Six Sigma since 1999. Six Sigma is an approach that is used in industry to methodically solve problems, and I've used Six Sigma to solve countless problems in my career. I've also applied the Six Sigma thought process and approach in my personal life and it's helped me become the man I am today. I use Six Sigma tools and techniques to transform men's lives and their families through my coaching business, Change YOUniversity.

Six Sigma is in my DNA. I'm a problem solver. Big problems inspire me, and the methodical data-driven approach to solving problems almost always uncovers a root cause that previously was unknown.

Duh….

Perhaps I should apply Six Sigma to this problem called cancer that I now have.

Duh…

I've avoided it because, truth be known, I didn't want to see the data. I knew the data would reveal survival rates and I didn't want to know the "number" that predicted my own survival rate. Once you hear a number about survival rate, you can never forget it, and it's permanently imprinted. The number invokes fear and the fear drives you crazy.

However, given that my cancer is of unknown primary source and this only occurs in between one and 10% of head and neck cancer cases[v], it would be foolish for me to let fear stop me from doing the research to uncover more details about this fairly rare occurrence called Cancer of Unknown Primary Source (CUPS).

• • •

We were poor growing up. I remember Christmas and my friends sharing they'd gotten tons of new toys (remote controlled cars, digital alarm clocks, skis…), all the things that I never got. Instead of extravagant gifts, mom always made sure we had one or two heartfelt gifts. I was jealous of my friends. But I had something they didn't have. I had a small metal box filled with parts from gadgets I'd torn apart and rebuilt. When I was bored, I'd pull out that box and rebuild an old alarm clock that somebody had thrown in the trash, or I'd take apart a remote controlled car that we'd bought at a yard sale for $1 and I'd find the wire that had come unsoldered causing it to malfunction. I'd plug the soldering iron in, re-solder the wire, put batteries in, and vroom…the RC car was as good as new.

Euphoria. There's no other way to describe the feeling I got after fixing something that somebody else had thrown in the trash. I remember mom needing a dishwasher and finding one for $10 at a yard sale. I ripped it apart, found the problem and mom used that dishwasher for the next 20 years!

When I was 15 years old, I was mowing a lawn for extra money. I looked on the side of the garage and I saw a pile of motorcycle parts. After mowing, I asked about it. "Oh, that's my old Honda CB 160. It was made in 1967. We tore it apart to try to fix it but were never able to fix it, so we just put it in a pile."

My heart started racing. 1967 was the year I was born, and I wanted a motorcycle to ride when I turned 16 but we couldn't afford to buy me one.

"Can I buy it?" I asked.

"No. But if you promise to put it together and get it running, I'll give it to you."

"Deal!" I said.

That summer, while my friends were at the beach, I was in my backyard working on that motorcycle. When they called me and asked me to go to the movies, I declined. I wanted to work on my motorcycle. I'd spend hours hand sanding the frame or tearing the carburetor apart and rebuilding it. I bought primer and red spray paint and my brother and I painted it in my shed. He's an artist and he painted flames on the gas tank!

As I methodically rebuilt it, I was ecstatic to see if it would run. Finally, the day arrived. I put gas in the gas tank and got ready to start it. Unfortunately, the kick starter had stripped out and it couldn't be fixed without tearing the engine apart. Fortunately, it had an electric start as well. I didn't have a battery for the bike (I couldn't afford it), but I did have jumper cables. I attached the jumper cables to the battery wires, pushed the electric start button, and it fired up!

Wahoo! It works, it works, it works! I was ecstatic. My brother and I high fived each other. I'd taken a basket of parts that were once a motorcycle that someone else couldn't fix and I fixed it.

This pattern of fixing things continued with my first car, my second car, my second motorcycle, and a third motorcycle that also started as a box of parts.

My problem-solving mind helped me identify a path to college through scholarships that I earned because I analyzed the factors that contributed to other people who had won scholarships. I put these factors into my life (leadership as class president, vice president of Spanish club, volunteering, etc.), and I won more scholarships than anyone else in my class. These scholarships enabled me to be the first person in my family to attend college.

Can you guess what my degree was in? Engineering, of course! One summer after moving to Seattle, I decided I wanted an internship in engineering. I put my problem-solving brain to work. I went to the job center and I found a job opening at Sundstrand Data Control. I knew a simple resume wouldn't be sufficient to get me the job, so I put my problem solving brain to work. I identified a cryptic signature at the bottom of the job opening. I found the nearest payphone, called Sundstrand, and asked for Bob, the hiring manager.

To my shock, Bob answered the phone. He asked about me and I told him about my passion for solving problems. I shared the story of the CB160. He was fascinated. He asked me to come in. A few days later I was making $11 an hour as a summer intern for Sundstrand Data Control in Redmond! That was a ton of money considering the most I'd made was minimum wage prior to that—$3.85 per hour in those days.

That job paid for my college and turned into my full-time career after graduating. That job sent me to Six Sigma school and helped me earn my Master Black Belt in Six Sigma. I learned how to solve manufacturing problems and earned many awards for my problem-solving skills.

That job also opened up my next job at Microsoft. I'd trained an individual in Six Sigma at Sundstrand and he moved to Microsoft. When a Six Sigma job came open at

Microsoft, he called me up, I got the interview, and I was hired!

Microsoft gave me the opportunity to solve some massive problems. The largest being the Xbox 360 three-flashing-lights problem. I'm not going to share the gory details here, but suffice it to say that my Six Sigma problem-solving skills quantified and predicted the billion-dollar warranty impact. More importantly, however, my Six Sigma skills helped dramatically improve manufacturing yields and eliminate the "bone pile" of hardware that was previously not repairable, earning me another award.

I used my Six Sigma skills to identify the root cause of the XBox 360 three-flashing-lights problem, and ultimately drive the solutions to this massive problem.

My cancer of unknown primary source reminds me a lot of the three-flashing-lights problem on Xbox 360. We didn't know what was causing the problem so we took a trip to the repair center. For confidentiality reasons, I can't share the details. However, I will say that we had very little data at the time to help us isolate the problem, so we had to rely on observation and experimentation for a few months to try to stop the problem even though we didn't know the root cause.

During this trip, I discovered some data. It was handwritten. This data identified the failure code for all Xbox 360s that came in. I used this data to focus the problem-solving team. I used the data to convince management to hire resources to help me compile more data.

Together with my team, we were able to pinpoint the exact problem and identify other problems that were previously unknown. We used this data to eliminate the three-flashing-lights problem. At the time, it was the biggest problem I'd ever solved.

There's one very important detail that I left out. After we had the data, we didn't know how to analyze it. We spent a few months and were still unable to analyze the data to isolate the problems. I knew we needed to find an expert.

I used my problem-solving skills, and after giving a keynote address at a data conference, I flew to North Carolina to talk with my friends at SAS, the company that makes JMP, the statistical analysis tool I use to analyze data. My friend Brad (who built the experimentation platform in JMP) quickly said, "You need to use Kaplan Meier."

Duh….

Of course, I needed to use Kaplan Meier.

"Um, Brad…what's Kaplan Meier."

"It's a statistical technique that was developed in the medical field to measure survival rates of cancer patients."

"How do I learn more?"

"Bill Meeker is the expert. I'll introduce you."

On the plane ride home, I taught myself Kaplan Meier. I applied it to the data that we were previously unable to analyze, and almost immediately, I saw patterns that we never saw before. We quickly started identifying problems and implementing fixes that we had been unable to see before.

Bill Meeker helped us quantify the overall impact and taught me the details of Kaplan Meier.

Today, the quality levels for Xbox 360 are the best in industry. Many of the tools and techniques that I introduced are being used to achieve these quality levels.

I'm a problem solver.

It was now time to apply my problem-solving skills to the biggest problem I've ever faced: cancer.

Cancer of Unknown Primary Source. In manufacturing, we called this NFF (No Fault Found), and it was the biggest driver of return costs. By far, NFF was the hardest to diagnose as well.

My cancer is NFF.

I got to work immediately and began researching. I'd use the same techniques to solve this problem as well. I'd need to find some data, I'd need to analyze it statistically, I'd need to identify the world experts, and I'd need to be relentless until the problem was solved.

Within a few minutes, I discovered that CUPS was a one to 10% problem. I found a PowerPoint from UCLA that talked specifically about CUPS. And I found the Kaplan Meier survival rates comparing treatment for Cancer of Unknown Primary Source (CUPS) with Cancer of Known Primary Source. As expected, the survival rates were significantly lower for CUPS than for known primary source.

> *"Nothing focuses the mind like a firing squad."*
> — Napoleon

I dug deeper into the data and I discovered that a new approach was able to identify the source of cancer for 72% of patients with Cancer of Unknown Primary Source. 72%! This new approach had a high likelihood of identifying the source of my cancer! And if the source of my cancer could be identified, the treatment could be more targeted, and my chances of survival would certainly go up!

Pain drives change. I know, you keep hearing it, but it's true. The pain of not knowing the source of my cancer drove me to change and start doing the research. The research identified a new source of pain, lower survival rates. That pain is now driving me to change my approach to interacting with my oncologists and asking questions scientifically.

I dug up the original study[v], printed it, and pulled out my highlighter. Transoral Robotic Surgery (TORS) enables surgeons to perform surgery on the tongue that previously required the splitting of the mandible to perform. In this surgery of the tongue, surgeons were able to see and perform precise biopsies in areas that were previously inaccessible. Because of this, they were able to identify the source of cancer in 72% of the patients and remove it! Furthermore, a large portion of the source identified was BOT (base of tongue).

I looked closer at the report and realized the raw data was included (at row level detail for the geeks that are reading this!). I quickly imported the pdf data into Power BI and transformed it using Power Query.

Within a few minutes I began visualizing the data. I quickly realized that 74% of those in this study were males and the median age (56) was just a little older than I am (51). As I studied the data closer, I discovered that the actual size of the tumor that was identified in TORS was listed. The median size was .9 centimeters (a little smaller than an inch). No wonder they didn't locate the cancer (if it is on my tongue)! A random biopsy of the tongue to find a tumor .9 centimeters? Not very likely. Here's the Power BI report I pulled together:

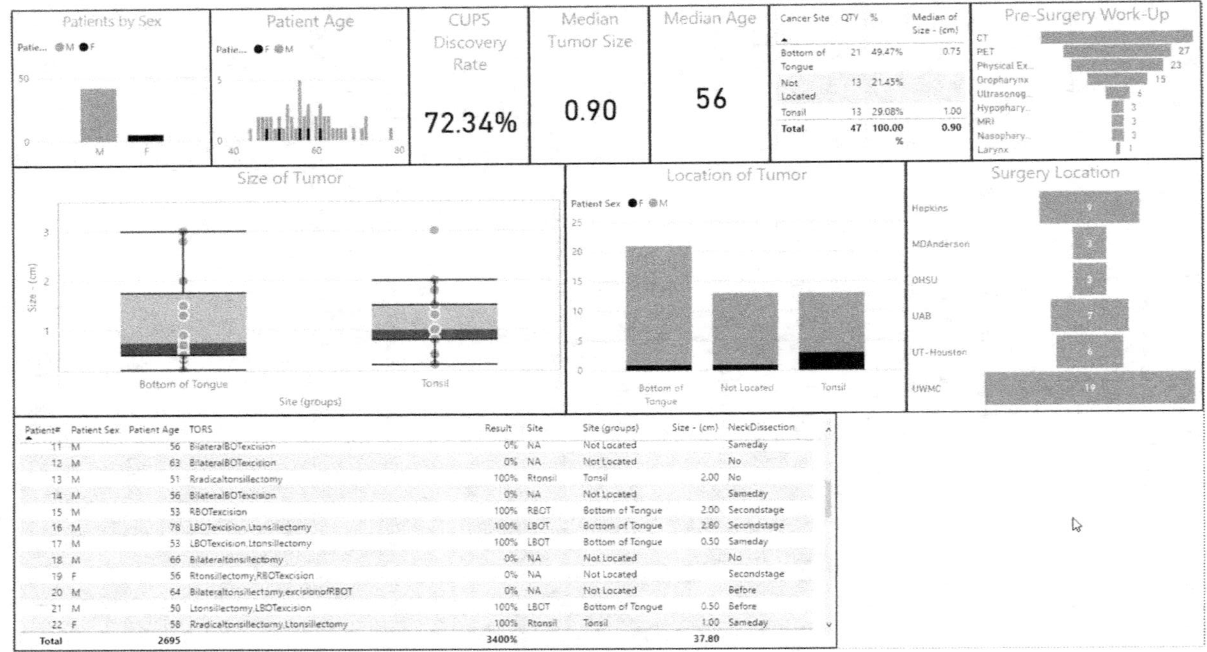

Cancer Site	QTV	%	Median of Size - (cm)
Bottom of Tongue	21	49.47%	0.75
Not Located	13	21.45%	
Tonsil	13	29.08%	1.00
Total	47	100.00%	0.90

Patient#	Patient Sex	Patient Age	TORS	Result	Site	Site (groups)	Size - (cm)	NeckDissection
11	M	56	BilateralBOTexcision	0%	NA	Not Located		Sameday
12	M	63	BilateralBOTexcision	0%	NA	Not Located		No
13	M	51	Rradicaltonsillectomy	100%	Rtonsil	Tonsil	2.00	No
14	M	56	BilateralBOTexcision	0%	NA	Not Located		Sameday
15	M	53	RBOTexcision	100%	RBOT	Bottom of Tongue	2.00	Secondstage
16	M	78	LBOTexcision,Ltonsillectomy	100%	LBOT	Bottom of Tongue	2.80	Secondstage
17	M	53	LBOTexcision,Ltonsillectomy	100%	LBOT	Bottom of Tongue	0.50	Sameday
18	M	66	Bilateraltonsillectomy	0%	NA	Not Located		No
19	F	56	Rtonsillectomy,RBOTexcision	0%	NA	Not Located		Secondstage
20	M	64	Bilateraltonsillectomy,excisionofRBOT	0%	NA	Not Located		Before
21	M	50	Ltonsillectomy,LBOTexcision	100%	LBOT	Bottom of Tongue	0.50	Before
22	F	58	Rradicaltonsillectomy,Ltonsillectomy	100%	Rtonsil	Tonsil	1.00	Sameday
Total		2695		3400%			37.80	

I've done this a thousand times in my career, but nothing I've done has been as important as this. The data convicted me that I needed to learn more about my procedure and ask if I'd had TORS. If not, why not? If so, what was revealed?

My meeting with the radiation oncologist was Monday. Fortunately, I'd called ahead and requested 30 minutes to discuss my case. We had a great conversation. I discovered that TORS was not performed. I asked why, and was told because the TORS robot was not available at the hospital that did the surgery. When she shared the certainty of the tumor team that my cancer was in the base of my tongue, I told her I agreed based on the data I'd found.

When I shared the Kaplan Meier plots comparing survival rates of Cancer of Unknown Primary Source vs. Known Primary Source, she agreed with my conclusion. Further evaluation via TORS was a wise and prudent decision.

She consulted her colleagues and they shared that UW and MD Anderson had TORS equipment. I shared the paper I'd found with her and discovered that UW had the most results. This gave me even more confidence that if I could get into the UW and get TORS, it would be done with a very experienced team!

She called the UW and referred me, reminding me that it might take a while to get in.

I didn't have a while. My life was at stake.

The next day I called the UW scheduling office. They gave me the phone number for the TORs surgeon's office. I called his assistant and left a message.

Today at 11:30 a.m., I heard back from her. It would be two weeks before I could see the surgeon. I apologized in advance for being a pain in the butt, but I shared that my request was urgent because radiation was scheduled to start in 12 days. She politely said, "Let me call you back".

Twenty minutes later, I received her call. She had talked to the surgeon and he said he would like to bring my case to the UW tumor board later that afternoon!

My jaw hit the floor. How is it that 48 hours ago I'd received the referral, and without a face-to-face appointment, had my case going in front of the UW tumor board?

I'm a man of great faith. I know how it happened. I have many people praying for me, and I firmly believe that God intervened on my behalf to get my case in front of the tumor board.

• • •

It's now 6:00 in the evening, two hours after the tumor board was to review my case. I haven't heard back yet, but expect to hear tomorrow. Furthermore, I'm extremely confident that they will decide to perform TORS on me because of the unique nature of my case.

Thank You, Jesus, for this miracle. Thank You for my ability to research and analyze data. Thank You for the discovery of TORS in my research, and thank You for the promise that this surgery has a high likelihood of identifying the primary source of my cancer. Thank You that You've created me to be a problem solver and given me the skills of data analysis. Thank You that I discovered the data and that the UW is just across the bridge from my home. Thank You for the scheduling nurse going directly to the surgeon today, and thank You for his willingness to bring my case to the tumor board. Thank You in advance for the promise that I will receive TORS and they will find my cancer. Lord, I pray my writing and my story will reach people who need hope. I pray it will reach people who have cancer but don't know it yet and it will inspire them to get that lump checked. Thank You, Jesus, for my family. Guide them and protect them through this journey.

Questions to Consider

1. What are your unique skills and abilities? How can you apply them to help you overcome your situation?

2. Have you identified an "expert" to help you? If not, why not?

3. How can I help?

7/18/2019

Wahoo!!

Sitting at UW. Just talked to the surgeon. Writing this from my app, so it will be brief.

I've been accepted and they are going to do the TORS surgery on me! Surgery is scheduled for August 2nd. My heart is beating out of my chest, I'm so excited. I feel like this is a miracle! (I don't use that term lightly; I really believe it is given the events that led up to this.) I will keep you posted on details as I get them.

Thank you everyone for your prayers and encouragement. I am heading out on my family's annual vacation.

By God's grace I have a solid plan for my treatment, and I will be resting and recharging in preparation for this next phase of treatment.

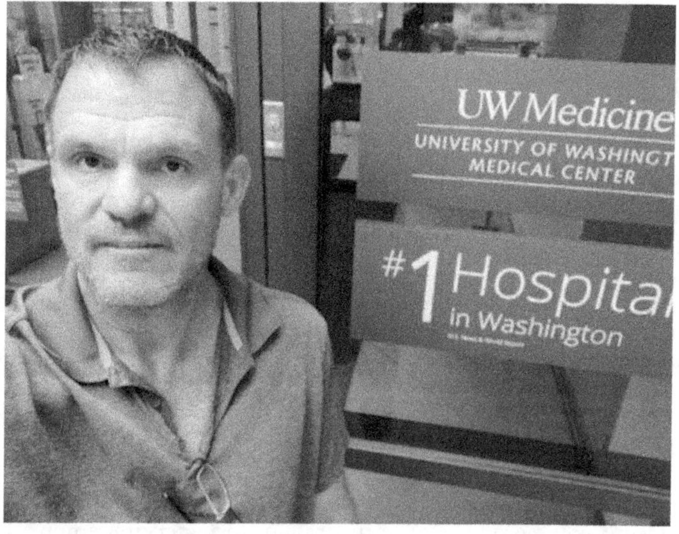
UW Medicine
UNIVERSITY OF WASHINGT
MEDICAL CENTER
#1 Hospital
in Washington

8/2/2019

The Mighty Hand of God

Sitting in the pre-op room and wanted to share a brief update.

Here we go! Transoral Robotic Surgery will begin at 7:30 a.m. PST and be completed by 9. It's been a series of what I truly believe to be small miracles getting me to the discovery and now surgery using TORS.

The doctor guesstimates 50/50 chance they will find the cancer.

Not me. I believe that I was guided here by the mighty hand of God.

He knows exactly where the cancer is, and He will guide the surgeon's hands as they guide the robot to find and completely and permanently remove the cancer!

All prayers are appreciated this morning. Thank you all for the constant encouragement. Stay tuned for the good news!

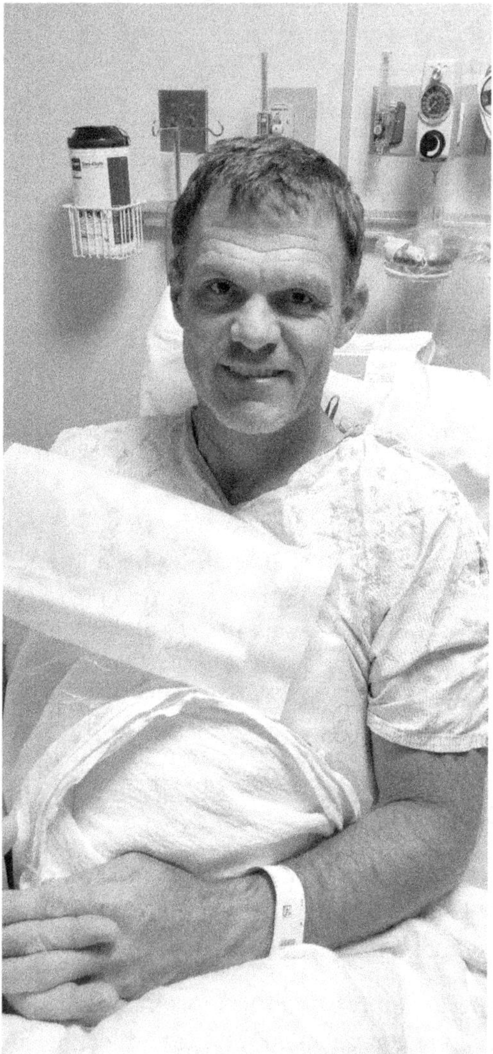

CHAPTER 9

8/2/2019

The Results Are In!

*Death and Life are in the power of the tongue and
those who love it will eat its fruit*
— Proverbs 18:21

A little more than 10 hours ago I was in the operating room. I looked at the surgeon and with 100% confidence, I boldly proclaimed this:

"You're going to find the cancer and remove it completely."

They responded by saying, "We'll do our best."

I repeated this to the nurses, doctors, and everyone else that was in the operating room with the Trans Oral Robotic Surgery Robot.

"You're going to find the cancer and remove it completely."

I know it sounds a little "woo woo," but I firmly believe that what we say and how we say it brings life or death (figuratively or literally). In my first book, I talk about how I used my words to transform me from the inside out. My counselor and friend taught it to me. It's called "mirror work" and it's a requirement for every man I coach. Literally, we help men define the man they want to be. Then we challenge them to speak these statements out loud while looking directly into their eyes in the mirror and speaking with such boldness that they absolutely believe it, even if the man they are isn't the man they want to be.

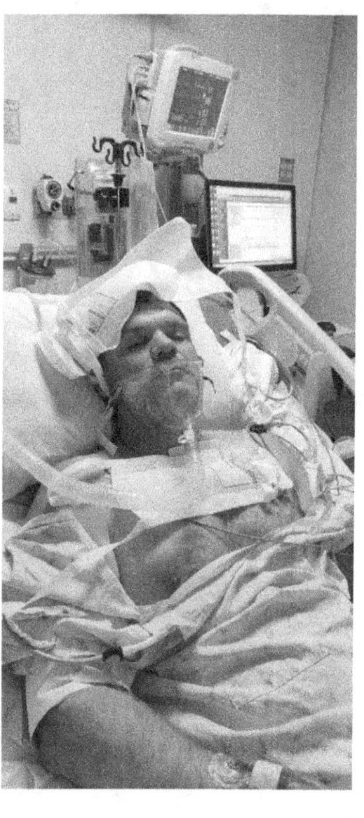

It transformed my life and it transforms their lives.

I've been speaking the same words with absolute belief since I discovered TORS—that they'd find cancer and completely remove it. A few days ago, I had nearly a dozen men lay their hands on me and boldly proclaim it as well. One man finished the prayer by saying, *"Jesus, the doctors may not know where the cancer is, but You do. Guide their hands and their eyes during surgery to find it and completely remove it."* Thank you for that bold prayer and belief!

But before I get to the results, it's very important to share the events of the last few weeks in a little more detail to fully appreciate how I got here.

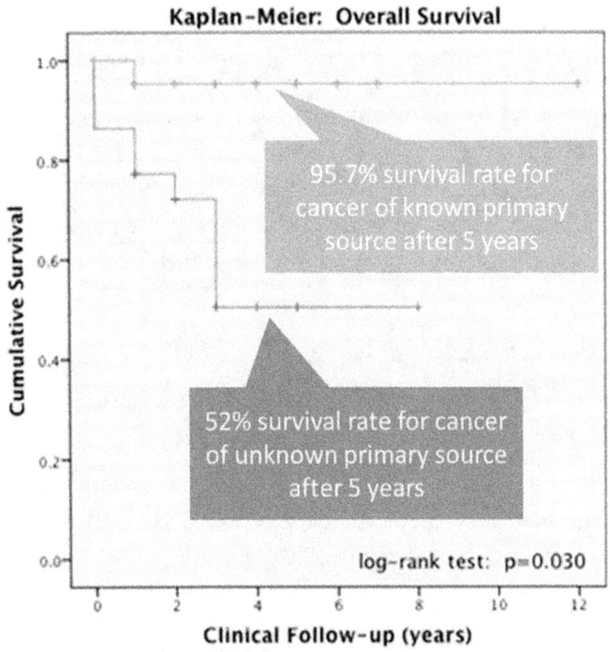

Recall I mentioned a little earlier that I came across a study that showed the survival rates for people with the exact type of cancer and location that I have. In the previous blog, I decided to protect my wife and family from the data I'd discovered, but I'm going to share it here using the previously mentioned Kaplan-Meier plots.

When I saw these plots[v], my heart dropped. For those who don't know how to interpret the plot, there are two lines. The first line represents head and neck cancer patients where they successfully identified and treated the primary source of the cancer. The second line represents people exactly like me—people where they were unable to identify the primary source for cancer. The survival rates are statistically different (p=.03 means there is a 3% chance of being wrong when stating the survival rates are different for cancer of unknown primary source than for cancer of known primary source).

The data representing my situation was clear and compelling. There was a 52% chance of survival after five years. Stated differently, I could flip a coin and the probability of it being heads was the same probability of me being alive in five years. However, because I understand Kaplan Meier, I knew it wasn't five years; it was two years.

I had a 52% chance of being alive in two years if I continued down the path that ALL of the professional doctors recommended at tumor board.

Let that sink in for a minute. It only took a microsecond for me to realize that I needed to take action on this data. Literally, my life and my family depended on it.

Pain drives change. It's the title of my first book and it will probably be etched on my tombstone. This statement will become part of my legacy. The pain of sticking my head in the sand and choosing to blindly accept the outcome was greater than the pain of me doing deeper research. I chose to research. My life depended on it.

One other brief note. I decided when I saw this data that I would NOT share it with my wife or my children. As a father and husband, I take my responsibility to protect my family very seriously and I chose to protect them from the fear that would ensue when they saw this data. My challenge to every man that is reading this is to ask yourself the question:

Am I protecting my wife and children or am I avoiding my God-given responsibility to do so?

If you are not actively protecting your family, it's time to man up.

Make a decision now and start protecting them!

If you don't know how, email <u>damon@changeYOUniversity.org</u>. I am actively coaching men in my coaching business and transforming generations in their family because they have decided to man up.

Man UP!

I know I'm being bold, but I won't apologize for it. The statistics are clear on the impact of a father in children's lives. You can read about this in Chapter 5 of my first book, *Pain Drives Change*. Man up and start protecting your family emotionally, physically, and financially. Your unborn grandchildren are dependent on your decision to do so.

• • •

Ok, back to my cancer story.

The data from the same article on survival rates also indicated that 72% of the time, Transoral Robotic Surgery identifies the primary source. If I could somehow get TORS, my likelihood of living had a high probability of shifting to 95% or higher!

My wife calls it hyper-focus mode. I call it a gift from God. When there's a problem to solve, it kicks in and I'm relentless until the problem is solved. Increasing the likelihood of being alive in five years to >95% was easily the biggest problem to solve of my life.

Study after study after study confirmed the findings: TORS is highly effective at finding CUPS in the base of the tongue. I knew I needed TORS and I'd stop at nothing to get it.

When I shared the Kaplan-Meier plots with my oncologist, she quickly got up, consulted her peers, and put an emergency referral into the UW. She cautioned me that it might be weeks before I would get in to see the surgeon. It was a risk I decided to take.

The next day, when I hadn't heard back from the UW scheduling department, I looked on the internet and found the phone number for UW scheduling. I called and they couldn't find my referral, saying it might not be in the system yet.

I said thank you, hung up, and immediately called back. This time the receptionist found something in the system. She gave me the direct phone number for the TORs surgeon's scheduling nurse. I said thank you and hung up.

I called the scheduling nurse and left a message. I didn't hear back.

The next morning, I woke up and I was anxious, praying fervently that I'd hear back from the UW. At 11:30 a.m., my cell phone rang. It was the scheduling nurse. She shared that the surgeon didn't have any openings and referred me to his other office. I thanked her, but kindly pressed her on the phone.

"I have cancer and my radiation is schedule to start in 10 days. Is there any way he could get me in earlier?" I pleaded.

She pulled up the calendar and was able to find a few openings, but I shared with her that I'd be on vacation in Eastern Washington on the dates she provided. I let her know, however, that I'd gladly drive the six hours to see him if possible.

"Let me call you back in a few minutes," she said.

Twenty minutes later, the phone rang.

"I just spoke with the surgeon directly. He'd like to take your case to the UW tumor board today at 4:00," she said.

Tears welled up in my eyes and I thanked her repeatedly for being my advocate.

"Unfortunately, we can't locate your records and they are all needed within an hour if your case is going to go in front of the tumor board."

"I'll make it happen," I responded.

I hung up my phone and searched for my nurse navigator's phone number. I couldn't find it. I searched for the phone number of Evergreen on my phone. I couldn't find it. I searched for the phone number of the other nurse navigator. I couldn't find it. I searched for the phone number of a consultant I was scheduled to have lunch with. I couldn't find it.

My phone numbers had literally been wiped from my phone and I didn't know what number to dial to talk with Evergreen to get my records to UW!

I prayed, called my wife, and she located the paperwork for my oncologist. I thanked her, hung up, and called my oncologist. The receptionist answered. She assured me that all paperwork of my case history would be there on time. I thanked her and asked her to confirm when it arrived.

Less than 30 minutes later, I received the call. UW had all the history they needed!

The next four hours, my heart raced out of my chest. I'd just experienced what I believe was a miracle.

Unfortunately, I didn't hear back from UW that day. The next day, my family and I were leaving on vacation for a week, and so I doubted I'd hear back for at least a week.

I was wrong. My phone rang at 9:00 a.m. It was the scheduling nurse. "Damon, how soon can you be here? We just had a cancellation."

"I'm on my way. I just have to drive across the bridge. See you in 40 minutes."

I called my wife and told her we'd just experienced another small miracle. I was so excited.

I was overwhelmed with the quality of care I received at UW and will be forever grateful to the scheduling nurse for making this visit happen.

The surgeon shared some background and said that there were basically three outcomes:

1. A grand slam. They could find it, remove it completely—including the margins—and it would be forever removed from my tongue.

2. Discover it. They could find it, but might be unsuccessful at identifying the margins, in which case he wouldn't know if it was all out.

3. Not discover it. There was a 50/50 chance that he wouldn't find it.

    a. He also shared that it was possible that cancer simply didn't exist in my body any longer, that my immunity system might have fought it off, but that we wouldn't chance it.

He also shared that he'd talked to the radiologist to determine if the radiation treatment would be different if he found it. Finding it would allow the Radiologist to target radiation and would be a great outcome.

He asked me what I wanted to do. I didn't hesitate. "Let's do it."

I proceeded to ask a few more questions.

"How frequently does CUPs happen?"

"About 3% of the time," he responded.

"Were the Kaplan-Meier plots I'd previously seen valid (i.e., were the chances of my surviving after five years 50% if they didn't find it)?"

He shared that the data in the plots was valid at the time, but since then they'd refined treatment and survival rates were comparable at between 90 and 95%.

He shared that this type of cancer is rapidly rising and the tumors are quite small (.9 cm as I reminded him of my research).

He shared that I'd be in the hospital for two to three days, but that my recovery would be three to four weeks, and I could expect full recovery.

I asked him if he was one of the pioneers of this surgery and he shared that he was.

I asked how many times he'd done the surgery. He shared that he couldn't remember, but likely in the hundreds.

My confidence was high.

"Let's do it!" I reaffirmed.

A few hours later we'd scheduled my surgery for a week after my vacation. I was going in for TORS!

And here we are, nearly 12 hours from the surgery. I'm sitting here eating a liquid diet. I have experienced almost no pain, and I feel like going for a bike ride! Fortunately, I brought my computer and I pulled it out to start writing.

As I write, I once again am experiencing the "flow state" that I often experience when writing about my experiences. I literally cannot type fast enough to get my thoughts out.

I awoke from the surgery at around 10:00 a.m. It took a little longer than expected. My first words, "Did you get it?"

"WE GOT IT!!!! It was on the right side of your tongue. We removed everything including the margins!"

"A grand slam!" I proclaimed, followed by a smug, "I told you so!"

My wife later informed me that they didn't even need to biopsy my tongue. They visually saw it right next to the location where my tongue was previously biopsied.

A miracle? Absolutely!

If the original biopsy had found the cancer, I would NEVER have had TORS surgery. I would have relied on radiation to burn it out and would be five days into radiation right now.

Greg's prayer was clearly answered. Jesus guided the surgeon's eyes to the exact spot my cancer was. And since they knew where it was, I didn't have to have a "hemi glossectomy (i.e., half my tongue). I only had to have a tiny tumor removed from the right side of my tongue. Because of this, I am literally experiencing almost no pain. I've been up and walked around the hospital many times. I'm eating a liquid diet and I'm writing this "in the moment."

Words will never describe what I'm feeling today. I woke up from bed this morning at 4:15 after barely sleeping all night, not knowing my future with cancer. Uncertain of my long-term viability. Uncertain of how I'd handle the uncertainty of never knowing the source if they didn't find it.

But I chose faith. I told my wife on the drive over to the hospital that they would find the cancer and we'd be rejoicing when I awoke from the surgery. My faith convicted me of this outcome. When I awoke from the surgery, I was quickly reminded of God's hand guiding me every step of the way and God's hand guiding the surgeons as they saw and easily removed this cancer from my body.

After hearing the news, I felt a deep need to worship Jesus. I turned on Pandora radio and the song "There will be a Day" by Jeremy Camp played. Tears flowed from my eyes as I remembered my mom in Heaven and I truly felt like she was my guardian angel, watching over me today.

The next song was one of my favorite worship songs, "Your Great Name." Tears flowed and I raised my hands to the heavens praising Jesus for saving my life and revealing this cancer.

My wife came over and I could barely speak the words, but I told her of the data that I hadn't previously shared. I told her that I wanted to protect her and didn't share that the survival rate was 50% after five years because I didn't want her to worry. I looked her in the eye and I said, "We've experienced a miracle today," and asked her to pray for me and thank Jesus.

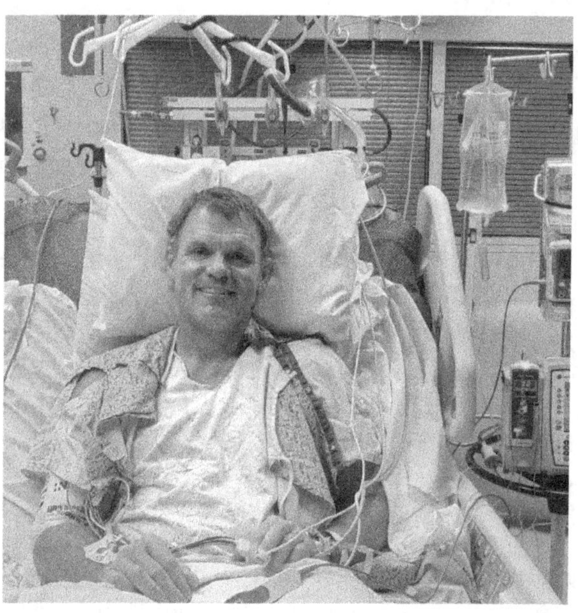

Thank You, Jesus, that You revealed my cancer to the surgeons today. Thank You for Your hand guiding my thoughts and decisions over the last few months, leading me to the miracle today. Thank You for the gift of life. Thank You for all the people who have been praying for me. Thank You for my children being so content that they rarely feared this cancer. Thank You for the men who laid hands on me and prayed. Thank You for my nurses today who are taking great care of me. Thank You for the

doctors that previously identified the cancer and thank You for the referral to the UW. Thank You for the gift of "hyper focus" that You have given me, the gift that has resulted in my body being cancer free as near as we know right now. Thank You in advance for the lives that will be impacted from my writing. I give You all the Glory Jesus.

Amen

Post Script: I just finished talking with one of the surgeons. He shared a few more details, saying "This is a good day." They identified the cancer using a camera. It was literally five mm from the location where my tonsils were removed six weeks ago. They were able to visually discern a difference and took a biopsy. The pathologist returned proclaiming it was cancer. He said everyone in the operating room high fived each other.

UW was one of the pioneers of this surgery 10 years ago, and today, they were celebrating another victory. He shared that TORS is becoming the "gold standard" for this type of cancer and that he is building his career on treating this form of cancer. He shared they will be bringing my case before the UW tumor board on Wednesday and deciding next steps, but typical protocol is "lightweight" radiation. He shared that the amount of radiation and the ability to focus the radiation because of this finding would be dramatically decreased.

He then said two things I'll never forget. The first was 10 years ago, this type of surgery wasn't possible. Removal of tumors like the one they'd found required splitting the mandible, a 12 to 15-hour surgery with significant degradation of quality of life afterwards. The second thing was that the next six years of my life will be dramatically improved because they found it versus if they'd had to proceed with radiation treatment when the source was unknown.

My family just left. We are celebrating. DAD BEAT CANCER TODAY!

Thank You, JESUS!

Questions to Consider

1. Do your words speak life? If not, why not?

2. Have you ever experienced a miracle in your life?

3. What can you celebrate today?

4. How can I help?

CHAPTER 10

8/27/2019

Emotion - The Gap Between Expectation and Experience

A little more than three weeks ago, I woke up from surgery and my first question was "did you get it?"

"We got it," the surgeon answered. Of course, I was incoherent, fell back asleep, and when I woke again, my first question was "did you get it?" "We got it," the surgeon answered. This time I remained awake.

They got it! They were able to visually see the cancer as a small lump in the right-hand side of my tongue, take a quick biopsy, and high-fived each other after it showed positive. The TORS robot, guided by the surgeon's hands, removed portions of the right-hand side of my tongue, and successfully removed all the cancer. The pathology would later show that the tumor was just 12 millimeters in size and was only five millimeters from the "blind" biopsy that was performed on my tongue just six weeks earlier.

Barely 12 hours after the surgery, my emotions were at a peak. I was elated and filled with energy because of the results. I pulled up my phone and I shared an emotion-filled Facebook Live broadcast sharing the news. I exuberantly declared that it was a miracle. A few short minutes, later I typed the previous chapter of this book.

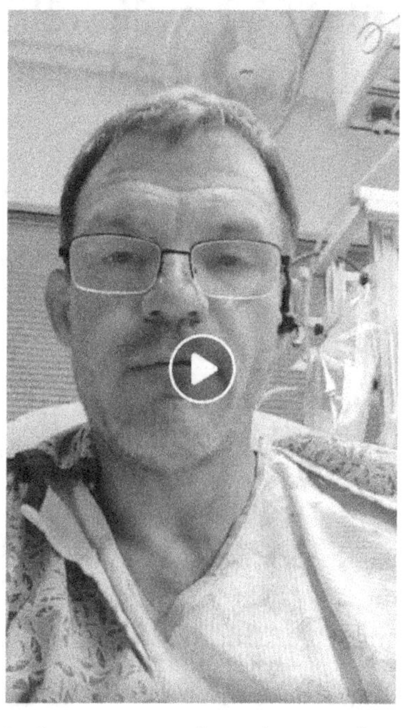

A few short weeks later, my emotions of elation quickly changed to confusion, anger and frustration after my fol-low-up visit with the doctor and radiation oncologist.

Before I share the results of the visit, I want to share a story that will help bring some clarity.

As a kid I loved to fish. I remember walking miles to toss my line in the water in hopes that I'd land a fish. I remem-ber going salmon fishing in the ocean and catching a few of those monsters. I remember going fishing with Monica when she was a kid and watching her bring in fish after fish after fish while others just watched. I wrote a blog about it years ago. It's true; fishing creates memories that last a lifetime.

Last year was Nathan's 10th birthday. I knew I wanted to start doing "man things" with him, but I didn't know what to do. To make a long story short, we went fishing in Canada with a man who has become one of my closer friends. The trip was incredible. I'll never forget the smile on Nathan's face when we landed the first king salmon. His primal yelp expressed how elated he was with the king salmon he successfully netted. You might say he was as excited to net that fish as I was to discover that my cancer had been successfully removed.

Emotion=Expectation minus Experience

Our emotions were high because the experience of catching and netting the king salmon exceeded any expectation he'd had. Prior to this trip, the largest fish he'd caught was only a few pounds, so subconsciously his expectation was "a little bigger than the trout we'd caught." His experience of catching and successfully netting a king salmon that weighed over 18 pounds dramatically exceeded his experience, so his emotions were very high, invoking the primal yelp!

After that trip, I decided that this trip to Canada with my son would be an annual occasion. The memories we build together are memories that I will cherish for the rest of my life. Unfortunately, the trip this year overlapped with my planned radiation treatment and I was afraid I'd have to cancel it. However, with the discovery of TORS and the surgery, I wouldn't be in the middle of radiation treatment. In fact, I'd be 10 days from my surgery and recovered enough to fish! We were going fishing!

We left the house early Wednesday morning and picked up my father-in-law. We had a great trip and caught a lot of salmon (3 kings each plus a couple of coho). The limit for kings is four per person and we wanted to limit out, so

Nathan and I decided to go out Saturday afternoon before our scheduled departure on Sunday. Grandpa was tired so he stayed back.

That morning we were fishing, and I noticed a lot of the other boats catching fish, but we failed to get even a hit. As I watched them net the fish a little closer, I noticed something that I hadn't seen before. The people catching the fish were locals, and they knew the tricks to catching salmon there. As I looked a little closer, I noticed that the leader on their poles 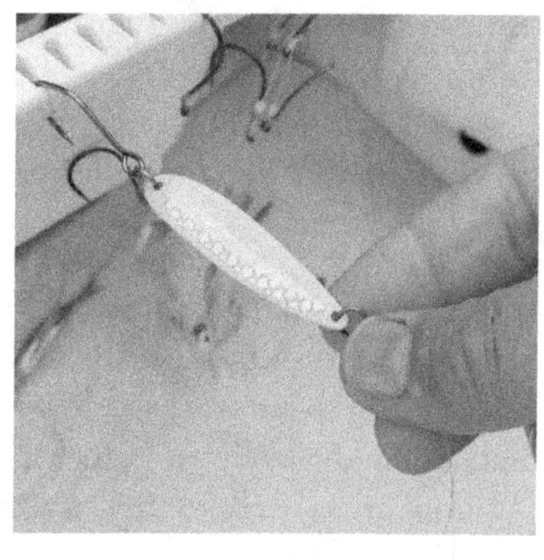 was at least twice as long as the leader we were using, and nearly twice as long as the leader recommended by the manufacturer of the flashers we used to catch fish.

I asked the camp host (who fishes every morning and catches a ton of fish) if my observation was correct.

"Absolutely," he said.

I was confused. I asked him to show me his fishing setup. I was always told to use 30″ of leader by virtually everyone that traveled to fish in Canada, but I stared at his pole with 72″ of leader. He was even using the same lures that I was using. The only difference was the leader length.

I was convinced and I asked him if he had any extra leader. He pulled out the 25# test and cut me off two pieces that were 75″ long, leaving me enough leader to tie the knots.

"Where should I go?" I asked him. He pointed to a spot barely five minutes from camp.

"Are you sure? I have fished for hours there and I've been skunked." I asked.

"Absolutely. I catch a ton of fish with this setup over there."

I decided to trust him. He was the expert and he had proof that his technique and his location were landing fish.

We drove across the water, rigged both poles with the longer leader, and dropped them to the exact depth he'd recommended.

Truth be told, I didn't expect that we'd catch any fish, but I relished the time on the boat with my son. He's become quite a fisherman and an expert netter, netting a lot of fish that would have been lost if not for his skills. In two years of fishing for kings he'd only lost one fish!

A few minutes after dropping our lines, I yelled "Fish!"

I quickly reeled this king in; he was easily the biggest fish I'd hooked since fishing up here. As the fish got closer to the boat, I told Nathan to grab the net. I saw the fish surface, and with a smile knew we'd bring him in the boat.

I was mistaken. The king turned his head and "spit the hook." Fish gone.

Our hearts were racing. We were both excited and saddened. "We'll get the next one," I shared with my son who was feeling a bit dejected because he wasn't able to net the fish.

A few minutes later, another fish was on. As I reeled this fish in, I told Nathan, "We'll get him." A few short minutes later this fish also spit the hook and we lost him.

"It's ok," I told Nathan, my heart thumping out of my chest. He let out a primal yelp, but this time it was a yelp of anger.

Emotion=Expectation minus Experience

Our experience over the last two years was that almost every fish we hooked we netted and brought into the boat. Our experience now was that we lost two in a row (this had never happened). Our emotions were high because our experience of netting fish was significantly lower than our expectation.

We dropped the line in again. Our hearts were racing as we knew this new technique of longer leader was working. We were hooking fish while all the other boats watched, wondering what was different.

A few minutes later, another fish on. A few minutes after that, another fish lost. A few minutes later, yet another fish on, and another fish lost at the boat.

Emotions increased as the excitement of hooking fish exceeded any experience we'd had before (four fish in less than 20 minutes!). Emotions decreased as we were unsuccessful at netting the fish.

We took a pause. A friend boated by and asked if we were using a single hook. "Yes" I responded. "Put a triple hook on; it will ensure they stay hooked."

I took a few minutes, modified our lures, and dropped them in.

A few minutes later, I watched the line pulling from the reel. This fish was HUGE.

"We're going to get him, Nathan. I'm going to play him out and wear him out." I wore him out.

He came to the edge of the boat and we saw him. Easily the biggest fish I'd seen—I'm guessing 25 to 30 pounds.

"Get ready," I told Nathan. The fish ran a little under the boat and I reeled him back up. Nathan started to net him, but I said "not yet. He's not tired. We'll get him."

The fish ran to the back of the boat and got tangled in the cable of the downrigger that had broken earlier in the week. A second later, the line came loose. Our monster king was lost.

I slammed my fist into the seat of the boat and watched my son wail in tears. He took responsibility for losing these fish and was crushed.

I placed him on my lap and hugged him as he cried and cried and cried. "We had him dad. It's my fault."

I gently looked him in the eye and reassured him that it wasn't his fault. We'd learned a new technique of fishing that more than doubled the leader length. Our net wasn't long enough to scoop the fish and as a result, when we got the fish to the boat, he wasn't able to get the net low enough to bring the fish in like he had earlier.

Emotion=Expectation minus Experience

My son's tears indicated the magnitude of his emotions. His expectation was that he'd net those fish, but his experience was that we lost five in a row.

He looked up from his tears at the flasher on the pole where we'd lost that fish. "Dad, the leader knot failed!"

He was right. It was a failure of the leader knot. The failure was mine. I'd tied the knot and it failed.

"It's my fault son. You did great."

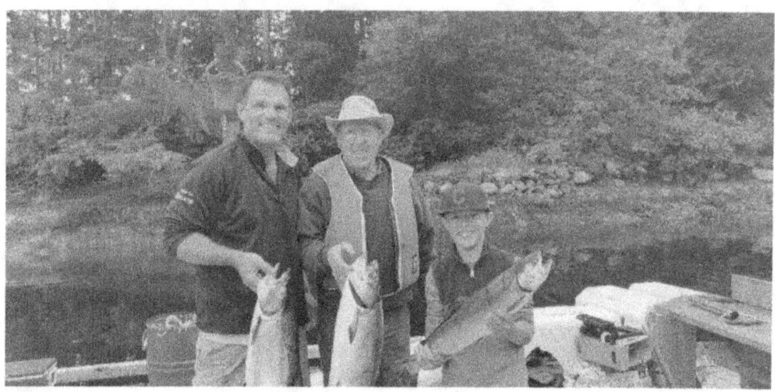

That was the last fish we hooked on the trip. I dreamed about hooking fish that night. Every day that I see friends post pictures of fish they caught brings up the emotion of losing those fish. Still, I'll never forget the lessons my son and I learned during those 45 minutes of fishing and hooking five fish and later losing them. And I had no clue that those same lessons would guide my decisions over the coming week to help me fight cancer.

Lesson #1:

<u>Emotion=Expectation-Experience.</u> We were ecstatic with hearts racing after hooking five fish in 45 minutes. Our experience exceeded any expectation we had. We were deflated and discouraged after losing all five fish because we'd only lost a few fish in the prior years. Our experience was less than our expectation.

Lesson #2:

<u>Ask an expert</u> - If you want to catch fish when others aren't, ask an expert who has experience catching fish. When we asked the expert, he told us to increase the length of our leader, a counter-intuitive action that was supported with data (lots of fish). We hooked five fish in 45 minutes because we listened to the advice of the expert.

Lesson #3:

<u>Different techniques require different equipment</u> - Our net handle was four-feet long; our leader was six-feet long, making it virtually impossible for an 11-year-old boy to net the fish. If we want to catch the fish, we need to get a different net.

Lesson #4:

<u>Emotional experiences bind us closer with those we love</u> - I'll never forget holding my son as tears streamed from our eyes. Our fishing trips, and this experience in particular, have built a bond that will last forever.

Lesson #5:

<u>Little details have a huge impact</u> - I was negligent with the knot I tied that ultimately failed resulting in losing the fish. If I'd redone the knot when I noticed it was fragile, we would have caught the fish. Instead, we lost it.

• • •

Now let's get back to my cancer story.

The surgeon tried multiple times to reach me while in Canada, but was unsuccessful. Unfortunately, he was on vacation during my follow-up appointment last Monday (the day after returning from fishing). His nurse practitioner shared the results of the pathology with me.

"Great news! Your pathology came back and they removed all the cancer with clear margins!"

I was elated, but it only lasted a brief moment.

"Unfortunately, the pathology shows that the type of cancer is different than the cancer they found in your lymph nodes. It's HPV negative."

"Unfortunately, the surgeon is on vacation and I don't know what it means," the surgeon's assistant shared.

Ouch. These words pierced my soul like a sharp sword. HPV positive is "very treatable." HPV negative is "not as treatable." HPV negative might indicate that they did NOT find the primary source of my cancer as I'd hoped and believed prior to this visit.

My mind raced. I couldn't fully celebrate the removal of the cancer because of the uncertainty associated with the pathology result.

Emotion=expectation minus experience. My expectation was that I'd hear that it was found, removed, and that I was cancer free. My experience was that they'd found and removed cancer, but it might not be the primary source of my cancer. It might be ANOTHER cancer. I experienced emotions of sadness, grief, confusion, and frustration.

"Maybe I'll get some answers in a few hours," I thought after my visit with the radiologist.

Once again, I was mistaken.

My expectation going into the radiologist was that I'd hear that my radiation treatment would be significantly reduced because they found the source. I was mistaken. The radiation treatment would be very similar to the original treatment plan, but a little more targeted to the side of my tongue where the cancer was found.

I couldn't hide my frustration. "This makes no sense! My surgeon said my treatment would be dramatically different and my quality of life would be significantly better. You're telling me something different."

"He's the surgeon. He shouldn't be giving radiation advice."

I became infuriated. "With all due respect, I am uncomfortable with your recommendation," I stated.

"I understand," she responded, "but unfortunately, there are a lot of different camps on how to treat this cancer."

I then asked her about the HPV negative pathology result. "It makes no sense to me, either," she responded.

I left her office angrier and more frustrated than I've been in years. My experience with the radiologist was dramatically different than the expectation I had from the surgeon, and my emotions were raging because of it.

I vented on my wife for a while, then I called a friend and vented.

I needed to take action. When I wasn't catching fish in Canada, I asked the expert who was catching tons of fish, and because of this I started hooking a lot of fish. I immediately scheduled an appointment with an expert, the radiologist at the University of Washington who specializes in head and neck cancer, particularly individuals who had TORS. My appointment would be a week later.

When I returned to work, people asked how I was doing. Unfortunately, I couldn't say "great" because of the newly discovered uncertainty.

I received the phone call Friday right before I went home. It was the UW.

"We just got the pathology results back from the re-screening of your tumor. They made a mistake. The tumor that was removed from your tongue was also HPV positive."

Wahoo! I high fived my son who was with me at work and my co-worker. I didn't expect the call, and the experience of the call exceeded any expectations I had. I was elated!

I just returned from my radiology appointment at the UW this morning. Much like the expert taught me how to catch fish, this expert revealed how to effectively treat head and neck cancer and dramatically improve my quality of life because the tumor was found and removed.

"I have one burning question," I asked the radiologist. "Is your treatment plan different because they found the cancer?"

He chuckled, "Of course it is!"

I asked him to explain.

"When you have a rat in a barn, you don't burn the whole barn down to kill the rat. You find where the rat lives and you target that specific area to kill it. Because we know exactly where your cancer was, we will target our treatment.

Your quality of life will definitely be better because we located the cancer."

I let out a sigh of relief. His answer was consistent with the surgeon's answer. Much like the expert in Canada told me how to fish (and it was different than the advice from people who only fish once a year), the experts in head and neck cancer told me exactly how to treat this cancer (and it was different than the radiologist who occasionally treated head and neck cancer).

He explained that my treatment would be a very light dose on the left side of my neck, a little higher dose on the right side, and a targeted dose around the right base of my tongue where the cancer was removed.

"This is very specialized treatment," he said. "It's important that you get treated by a specialist because patients who get similar treatment in non-specialized clinics drop out about 33% of the time."

"Why is that?" I asked.

"Because the level of care isn't available. The pain levels become intolerable and they quit. We have a lot of capabilities here that non-specialized clinics don't necessarily offer, and our treatment is very refined so we minimize the amount of pain that is induced from the radiation treatment."

Much like my lesson from the failed knot in Canada, the little details make a big difference. This radiologist specializes in treating this specific type of cancer and because of this, he "catches a lot more fish" (e.g. people finish their treatment and as a result survival rates are higher).

"What are the long-term effects from this treatment?" I asked.

- Your pain will be the same or greater than you just experienced starting at week three and peaking near the end of treatment. It will taper off one to two months after treatment.

- You'll have saliva loss. At six months it will be about 70%. Long term it will be 80%-90% returned. You'll barely notice it, but you might have to have water with you.

- You'll lose your taste for a while. Thanksgiving and Christmas meals won't be enjoyable, but Easter will be almost back to normal. You might have some loss of taste for sweets permanently and you might struggle to swallow breads and dry foods.

- You will have treated the cancer in the best-known method and have confidence that there is less than a 10% chance that it will return.

"What about not radiating. What are your thoughts?" I asked.

"It's a coin toss. About 20% of the time it returns without radiation. I've had patients not treat and return with no cancer and I've had patients not treat and return with cancer, but in a different location where we can't treat it. It's really up to you."

My wife and I looked at each other and we both had a level of confidence we didn't experience the previous week at the previous radiologist.

"Avoiding radiation is not an option. When can we start?"

"We'll get you fitted for a mask in two days and start 13 days after that," he said.

"Thank you," I said as I firmly shook his hand. "My confidence is dramatically higher than it was a week ago. I feel peace knowing that you specialize in head and neck cancer."

"How many people have you treated after TORS?" I asked.

"Hundreds," he said.

Much like the expert in Canada had caught dozens of fish while others were skunked, my expert would treat me with the specialized techniques that others simply aren't aware of because they have never treated cancer after TORS surgery. And my results will be similar. I'll be free of 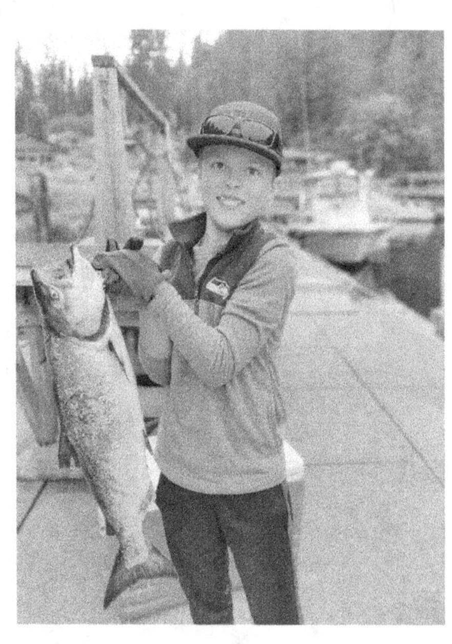 cancer with minimum impact to my quality of life.

Tears formed in my eyes on the drive home as I talked to my wife. "God is with us, dear. It's a miracle that we discovered TORS, it's a miracle that they found it, and we now have a radiologist who we fully trust to completely eradicate any remaining cancer cells from my body. I'm overwhelmed with gratitude; I think the emotions are going to start now that we have a solid plan in place."

Thank You, Jesus, that You revealed TORS to me. Thank You that You revealed cancer to the surgeons. Thank You that they removed it. Thank You that You prompted me to get a second opinion. Thank You for the treatment plan that doesn't require "burning the barn to kill the rat." Thank You for the hope I feel that this cancer will finally be gone for eternity. Thank You for my wife and her support. Thank You for my job and the support from my family, friends, and co-workers. Thank You for the lessons You taught me on the fishing trip with my son, and thank You for my family.

Questions to Consider

1. Do you have a child? What do you do with him or her to form special memories for a lifetime?

2. Are you 100% confident in your "plan" to solve the problem you are facing? If not, have you considered seeking additional "experts?"

3. How can I help?

CHAPTER 11

9/10/2019

Build a Bridge

....I reach my hands out to the heavens, yeah,
And I lift my voice to You alone.
To You alone...
And I sing Hallelujah, You are my God.
Maker of the heavens....
— Jeremy Camp

have a confession to make. I'm struggling. I'm really struggling. As I sit in the waiting room preparing to do my "dry run" for radiation that will start tomorrow, I'm struggling. Cancer sucks and I really, really, really don't want to do six weeks of radiation with a lifetime of side effects. My mind simply will not accept that I'm going to start radiation tomorrow. I try to make up every excuse I possibly can to avoid it.

When people ask me how I'm doing, I joke about them strapping my head to the radiation table, using the "mask" so that when the flesh that is getting scorched with the radiation to my mouth and neck, I won't move. The smoke will just come out my ears and they'll know they've cooked me enough to get the cancer out.

I guess I'm still in denial. I just came back from the dry run. I walked through the foot-thick lead door to my radiation "chamber" that is called "Discovery." Discovery. What an interesting name. Kinda like I discovered a lump on my neck just a little more than four months ago. Kinda like they discovered cancer in the lump with the needle through a biopsy. Kinda like they discovered another lymph node with cancer and failed to discover cancer in my tonsils after my surgery. Kinda like my discovery of TORS and the discovery of the 12 mm tumor in my right base of tongue because of it.

The next six weeks will be a journey of discovery for me as I discover how to intentionally expose myself to radiation that will kill any trace of cancer, which may or may not be present, and kill the cells that allow me to taste for a few months, with potential permanent damage to the cells that allow me to taste sweets and partial permanent damage to the cells that produce saliva in my mouth.

I entered the Discovery chamber and observed a very large mechanical device—the radiation machine.

"How are you doing?" the nurse asked.

I barely choked out the words as I fought the tears.

"I don't want to do this," I said.

A few minutes later, they put on my favorite Pandora radio station, Jeremy Camp Radio. I removed my shirt and they put a warm blanket across my chest. My neck laid across a plastic support and I placed the mold into my mouth that would keep my tongue from moving. They then laid the mask across my face and strapped me in. The mask holds my head firmly in place and I definitely can't move.

The large lead door shuts and they begin the "dry run." The motorized head of the radiation machine rotates around my head. I watch the aperture open and I see the reflection of a green laser on my mask. Precision placement is key, and the lasers will ensure that I'm in exactly the same location every day.

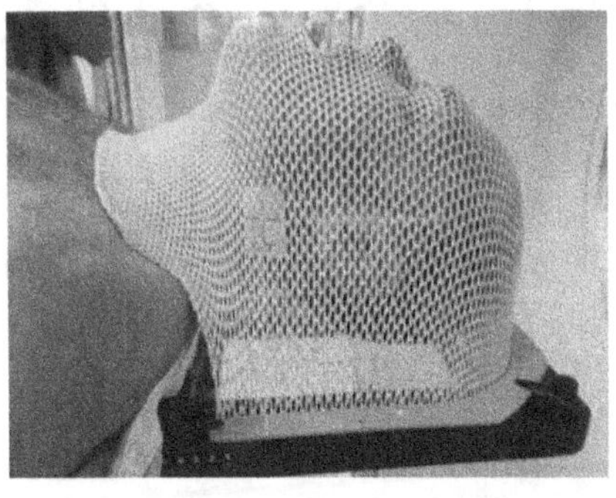

A few minutes later, I'm done with the dry run.

If you sense a bit of negativity and cynicism in my writing, it's because my writing is a picture into my soul. It's how I'm feeling. I try and try and try, and for some reason, I'm unable to push through this one. I feel a bit like a hypocrite because so many people come up to me and tell me how inspiring I am to them. They tell me how much courage I have.

I don't feel that way now. Honestly, I just want to run away from this and pretend it never happened. I tried to drown out my feelings by enjoying my favorite sweets for the last time. But the chocolate cake at lunch didn't satisfy my craving, so I had a cinnamon roll. It didn't work, either.

I miss you mom.

It was rare, but on the days that I felt like this, like I needed to cry and be held, you were there. You reminded me that it was ok, and you told me how proud you were of me. Your words inspired me and carried me through those days.

I miss you mom.

I'd do almost anything to hear your words today. "I'm proud of you son; you'll make it through this."

But I won't hear those words until I meet you in heaven. And I won't be meeting you in heaven for a very long time because I'm going to kick cancer's butt. I'm going to get through this season and I'm going to use my experience to inspire and encourage others who are struggling.

Stop whining, Damon.

Mom also used to say something else.

Build a bridge and get over it

So how do I get over it (my denial)?

By going through it. There's simply no other answer.

Debbie and I spent the weekend together alone. It wasn't like our normal date weekends. It was much different. My mood was somber. I cried and I whined. I shared my frustration and anger.

Exactly six years ago on September 10, 2013, Debbie told me she had cancer. The next two weeks were hell as the fear of death crept in. The words of the radiologist were very assuring. "It's the most treatable form of cancer on the planet." Radiation and chemotherapy would eradicate her cancer and we'd never have to deal with it again. And they did, until 16 months ago when Debbie told me she had another lump in the same place. This time surgery removed it and she's cancer free.

But why didn't the radiation kill everything? Why did she get another lump when her cells were cooked and poisoned from chemo? Why didn't radiation do the job on her?

And the big question that keeps me in denial: *If it didn't work for her then what confidence do I have that it will work for me?*

That's it. That's why I'm in denial. I don't see the purpose in radiation. The only purpose I see is that it's an "insurance clause" just in case there are still cancer cells. And these cancer cells could result in cancer in the future in a place where it might not be treatable.

I have a family to take care of. They need me to guide them and protect them. They need me to be there for them in the good times and the bad. Just like the phone call I got a few days ago when my daughter was sobbing. She needed her dad and I was there. Just like the conversation with my other daughter on her bed last night when she was sobbing. She needed her dad and I was there. My son needs me to model being a man of God so that he can be a man of God for his family.

I have a wife who I love with all my heart. A wife who needs me to be by her side as we navigate the waters of life.

This is why I need to have radiation. I'm not having radiation for ME, I'm having radiation for THEM. I might choose not to have radiation if it was just me. But it's not. I have a family that I love and I'm going to eradicate cancer from my body forever FOR THEM.

There's the bridge, mom.

I feel myself starting to get over it.

How selfish would it be for me to say, "I want to be able to taste sweets for the rest of my life so I'm going to put my family's security at risk?"

That's what it boils down to. My own selfish desires to continue enjoying sweets and be able to spit when I feel like it. My own selfish desires to avoid six weeks of pain. That's why I'm in denial.

Get over it.

Pity party or perspective, Damon? The pity party has been going on long enough. Now let's get some perspective.

- The three-year-old toddler resting his head on daddy's shoulders as he endures radiation. He's the one with courage.

- The man that my friend told me about who knew the radiation would blind him but it was necessary to save his life. He's the one with courage

- My friend who went through chemo for 14 months and stopped to enjoy life for a brief period that might ultimately cost him his life. He's the one with courage

- My wife who has endured cancer twice and has never complained about the side effects. She's the one with courage.

And I'm whining because I won't be able to taste sweets for the rest of my life and I'll be in pain for a few weeks.

Perhaps some cheese would go well with this whine.

Perspective is a powerful thing.

Get over it.

You have a family that needs you. You have people that you don't know that need to be inspired by your writing.

I've built the bridge and I feel like I'm getting over it. The bridge was perspective and purpose. And I'll get over it.

Thank You, Jesus, for perspective. Thank You for my family that will never experience the void of a dad who didn't survive cancer. Thank You for my wife whose courage through two rounds of cancer is an example for our family. Thank You for medicine that can eradicate cancer, and thank You for my home being less than 30 minutes from one of the top head and neck cancer treatment centers in the world. Thank You that my radiologist is considered one of the best for this type of cancer, and thank You that You made a way to find and remove the cancer. Thank You in advance for the lives that will be inspired as they read this and choose to take action.

And thank You, Jesus, for my mom. Thank You for her words that spoke to me even though she's with You. Thank you, mom. I needed you today and you were with me as I built this bridge.

Questions to Consider

1. Are you in denial?

2. What is the bigger purpose of you going through your struggle (i.e., the bridge to help you get over it?)

3. What are you thankful for today?

4. How can I help?

9/20/2019

I Can't

*"For God has not given me a spirit of fear, but of
power and love, and sound mind."*
— 2 Tim 1:7

just finished my 8th radiation treatment. That puts me at 26.7% complete. This is going to sound crazy, but stick with me....

I LOVE my daily dose of radiation!

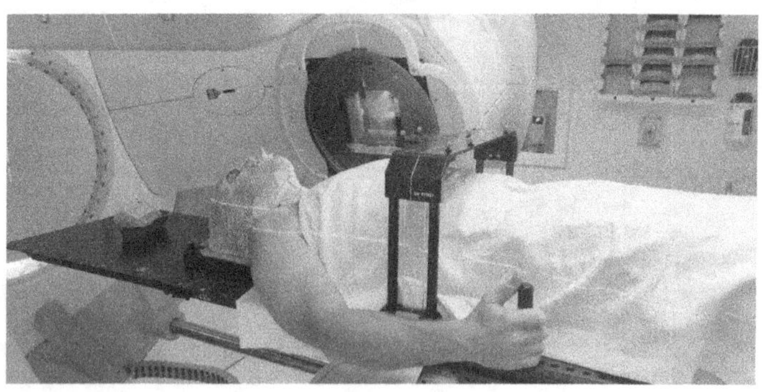

Don't get me wrong. I'm not looking forward to the pain, loss of taste, loss of saliva, and tiredness they are promising me. But I love my daily visits to UW for my radiation treatment.

Crazy, I know…and a lot different than my attitude a little less than two weeks ago where I was in denial and didn't want to do it.

What changed? Simple. My attitude and outlook. I chose action in lieu of my previous apathetic attitude toward radiation. Nothing else changed. Just my attitude and the resultant actions that followed.

What triggered this change? Pain. But not the pain of radiation treatment or cancer; it was the severe and debilitating pain I experienced more than 10 years ago. This pain drove me to change, and I'm still reaping the benefits of that change today.

In order to fully understand why I love my radiation treatments, I'll need to go back to that time when I was in extreme and debilitating pain.

It was January 17, 2007. The middle of "winter" in Seattle. Weeks of grey, rainy weather and no sign of the sun was getting me down. I called my wife on the phone, crying my eyes out. I was depressed and couldn't make it through the day. I was hopeless and miserable.

I'm bipolar and I was experiencing the depressive phase of manic depression. I'd been here before, but this time was different. I'd decided to stop taking my medication because it was killing my emotions (I felt like a zombie) and it had contributed to my massive weight gain (I was nearly 260 pounds with my ideal adult weight being 205 pounds). Stopping the medication helped me feel again. I certainly could feel my emotions now as I sobbed on the phone with my wife.

Two days later, I wrote in my journal. My depression had reached a point of debilitation.

"Stayed home from work. Couldn't get energy to get up"

I laid on the couch all morning with tears in my eyes, being overwhelmed with fear, anxiety, and depression. I felt hopeless. In my pain, I was forced to change. I called a friend and he encouraged me to go back on the medication. Reluctantly, I agreed.

My moods started to improve. Over the next few months, I started gathering clues about the cause of my depression. Here are a few excerpts from my journal:

January 23	...Feeling very sad and disheartened.... What is my future???
January 24	Moods fluctuate considerably within a day. Realized that I don't have a VISION...so nothing pulls me forward.
January 27	Feeling VERY sleepy and lethargic. Related to getting up at 5:30?
January 30	Third day in a row feeling good, wow! 10 minutes of sun lamp today, too.
February 5	Feeling more lethargic today. It is cloudy and gloomy out. Work is slow today as well...is that a clue?
February 6	Exercised at lunch yesterday, felt good.

February 16	Worked at home today. Felt good because I got some results (and watched a guy I'm mentoring get results).
June 7	Stopped taking Lexapro because feeling WAY too stimulated.
July 11	AWESOME Team Offsite. Developing leaders makes me PERFECTLY congruent.
Aug 15	Back to work after long vacation at Lake Roosevelt. Absolutely Incredible!

The "factors" that seemed to contribute to my depression (and/or help remove the depression)

- Having a vision for my future
- Getting adequate sleep
- Sunlight
- Exercise
- Mentoring/coaching
- Developing leaders
- Family vacation time

Unfortunately, a few months later, the weather began to turn, and I began feeling depressed again.

• • •

Before I share the rest of the story, I have a confession to make. I started writing this chapter almost two weeks ago and I haven't been able to finish it because I felt like a hypocrite writing about feeling AWESOME when it quickly became a lie.

I haven't been feeling awesome. I've been tired and consumed with something I didn't expect to happen. My body started to itch everywhere. I thought it was associated with the radiation, but the doctors swear it isn't. It got so bad that I woke up in the middle of the night scratching, but I found no relief. I called the dermatologist and, unfortunately, had to wait almost a week before seeing them. The itching became worse and worse. I became more and more frustrated and my calves were covered in sores where I'd scratched so much I broke through the skin.

And I'm writing a chapter about how great I feel? I simply couldn't do it. It was a lie.

When I finally met the dermatologist, I pleaded with her to do anything to stop the itching. She looked at my body and boldly declared, "I don't know what is causing this." She proceeded to take a biopsy declaring, "I doubt it will reveal anything, but we have to try." She then decided to throw everything at my itching to stop it. She prescribed creams and anti-itch pills and allergy medicine and moisturizers and….

But it didn't work. I woke up in the middle of the night and I itched so bad that I almost woke my wife up to take me to the hospital.

A few days later, I was watching my daughter's volleyball game and my arms began breaking out in little bumps everywhere. I quickly drove to the dermatologist's office only to find that they were closed. I called to talk with the on-call physician and got a voicemail.

The next morning, they called me back. "I'm sorry Mr. Stoddard, but there isn't anything more we can do. Are you showering regularly?"

"Yes!," I said.

"You might want to cut back on showers and make sure they are cold to lukewarm, and try not to use much soap."

"Oh, and did she tell you this would go on for weeks before it might clear up?"

"No, she didn't. Thank you for the call."

Weeks? I had to continue to deal with this itching for weeks? My spirits plummeted. Here I am going through radiation treatments for cancer and now I have to go through weeks of itching so badly that I am scratching through the skin?

> *Hope deferred makes the heart sick, but desire fulfilled is a tree of life.*
> — Proverbs 13:12

I was crushed. I became cynical and started snapping at my wife when she tried to have a conversation with me. My heart was sick.

I had a choice. I could dwell in my misery or I could accept it. I'm not sure when it happened, but I accepted it. My itchy skin was 100% out of my control. The specialists were doing all they could. I accepted it.

I continued doing everything I could to take care of myself, making sure I filled my time with things that gave me energy and removed things that didn't.

I had dinner with my friend and inspiration who is going through cancer that may be terminal. I rode my bike to and from work. I listened to worship music in my truck. I spent evenings coaching my junior football players. I spent an evening in the rain with my family watching our high school football team destroy their opponents. I went to the Casting Crowns concert with my family and worshipped my God who gives and takes away. I developed a program to help my coaches in Change YOUniversity grow to the next level. I spent time at my vacation home. I celebrated my being halfway done with radiation treatments by biking 20 miles in the sun along Lake Washington to my 15th treatment.

And somehow the itching doesn't consume me anymore. Maybe it's the medicine and the creams. Or maybe it's a result of continuing to love myself by taking care of myself that has almost eliminated my skin itching.

I just returned from the dermatologist. The biopsy was inconclusive. It might be weeks before my itching is completely gone. But it doesn't matter. I've accepted that I'll itch and I've accepted that we will never know what caused the itching. But it doesn't matter....

I just completed my 16th radiation treatment and I feel FANTASTIC. My energy is through the roof, the pain from the radiation only reveals itself when I swallow, and it's not extreme. I've lost my sense of taste and about half my saliva.

But I feel FANTASTIC.

Why do I feel fantastic? Let's go back in time to about 10 years ago when I learned a powerful lesson on life.

> *Your system is perfectly designed to get you the results you are getting...*
> — Deming

Fall was coming and I began to feel very anxious that once again, I was entering deep depression, the same depression that left me on the couch unable to get up and go to work less than a year earlier.

A few entries in my journal revealed some more clues as to why I was feeling depressed.

9/18/2007	Wellbutrin...started today.
10/03/2007	Woke up this morning and almost in tears for no reason...
10/06/2007	Going to start Lexapro today
10/08/2007	Debbie and I decided that the Lexapro isn't going to work...just makes me too distant. We're going to try to stabilize the Wellbutrin by going to SR vs. XL. Also, I'm going to stop being a victim...take walks in the morning, eat right, exercise, change my thought processes.
10/11/2007	Feeling REALLY sad and empty this morning....despair, no hope for the future
10/17/2007	Woke up anxious, called Dad and started to cry. Called Don and started to cry. Is this a spiritual battle?
10/18/2007	This is a spiritual battle, and I'm going to fight it with spiritual weapons! Tears again this morning. Began running in the mornings today.
10/19/2007	Feel better today than I have in a long time. Took 150 Welbutrin XL last night and 150 this morning. Attacking this like a spiritual battle. With HIM I will emerge victorious!

I'd decided to try a new medication to help with my depression—Wellbutrin. Unfortunately, the Wellbutrin didn't help my depression, so I started taking my old medication, Lexapro. A few days later I realized why I stopped taking the Lexapro. It numbed my emotions and it had a very negative impact on our relationship.

Debbie and I had the talk that would change my life and the lives of all the people I influence.

Apathy would say that I was a victim of bipolar and my family and I would suffer the consequences because of this biological condition. After all, I had a good excuse. I was born with bipolar and it was out of my control.

Action would say that I may not have control over my biological conditions, but I have complete control over my actions to minimize the impact.

Apathy or Action

I had a tough decision to make. Was I going to choose to remain apathetic about my condition or was I going to stop being a victim and take action? Pain drives change and I was suffering enormous emotional pain through my depression and anxiety.

I chose action.

> *"I'm going to stop being a victim...take walks in the morning, eat right, exercise, change my thought processes."*

The action I took started with a decision. A decision to start taking care of myself. A decision to start loving myself.

I wish I could say things got better after that decision. They didn't. In fact only three days later I woke up and wrote *"Feeling sad and empty this morning...despair, no hope for the future."*

A week later, nothing had changed. I was in tears and feeling helpless, full of fear and all alone. I called my dad crying my eyes out.

Then I called my pastor, my friend, and the man who has made a bigger impact on my life than anyone else.

"Don, I can't stop crying. I'm depressed, full of anxiety, and nothing is helping."

"Damon, I think it's a spiritual battle and you need to attack it spiritually. Read the book 'Waking the Dead,' spend time daily in the Bible, pray, and sing your favorite worship music."

The next morning was different. I woke up in tears again, but this time I wasn't a victim to my tears. I took action. I went for a run (well, actually it was a walk with a short jog in the middle), and during this run, I listened to my favorite worship music (very loud) and I verbally spoke a few of my favorite scriptures out loud.

2 Timothy 1:7

> *"For God has not given me a spirit of fear, but of power and love and sound mind."*

Wow, that felt good. So, I said it again, this time louder.

> *"For God has not given me a spirit of fear, but of power and love and sound mind."*

It was as if these words penetrated the fear and the anxiety and depression lifted. I stopped feeling like a victim and started feeling hope that I'd be victorious. So I said it again, this time I said it like I believed it!

> *"For God has not given me a spirit of fear, but of power and love and sound mind!"*

The next morning, I felt better than I had in a long time. My apathy was gone and now I was taking action.

> *"Attacking this like a spiritual battle. With HIM I will emerge victorious!"*

The next morning, I continued my routine and wrote in my journal "Feel Good." And the next morning I did the same and wrote in my journal "Feel Good." And the next and the next and the next…

Don was right. It was a spiritual battle, and for the first time in 40 years, I began winning the battle with my new spiritual weapons of scripture, worship music, time in nature, and taking care of my body by running!

But God was just getting started with my transformation. That weekend I attended a men's conference. I cried on the way to the conference but felt incredibly refreshed on the drive home. God gave me a vision for the purpose of my life at that conference. A vision that ignited a deep passion inside of me. A vision that would utilize everything I'd gone through for my entire life to benefit others. He gave me a vision for developing men.

> *"Without a vision the people perish."*
> — Proverbs 29:18

This new vision for my life inspired me. I no longer struggled to get out of bed in the morning, but began looking forward to my time in the morning to worship, exercise, and be in nature. To nurture the vision He'd given me while I was in the wilderness.

A month later I came across another scripture that explained where I was and where I'd be going.

> *"Blessed is the man who trusts in the LORD And whose trust is the LORD. For he will be like a tree planted by the water, that extends its roots by a stream and will not fear when the heat comes; but its leaves will be green, and it will not be anxious in a year of drought nor cease to yield fruit."*
> — Jeremiah 17:7-9

I was learning how to trust in the Lord. I was building deep roots. He was preparing me for the heat that would come into my life over the coming years, and He was showing me how not to be anxious in this heat and continue bearing fruit in my life.

12/22/2007	Sun lamp in the morning. I like how it makes me feel!
1/3/2008	Started training for a 5k today!
1/9/2008	Sunlamp or running or Wellbutrin are having a consistent effect on my attitude/moods
4/30/2008	Great meeting with my mentor. He pointed out that others are noticing I'm "changing" (e.g. considering others' needs before my own). God spoke to me in this moment.
6/02/2008	Good weekend. Been feeling pretty good for a long time

In the next few months, my relationship with Christ grew stronger than it had ever been. I set my alarm for 6:30 a.m. and every morning I got up. I stopped walking outside in the mornings because of the weather, but I started going to my chair in the living room. I discovered that I also suffered with S.A.D. (Seasonal Affective Disorder) and that using a sunlamp in the morning had the same impact on me that the sun did. I sat in front of the sunlamp, listened to worship music, read my Bible, and my soul was replenished.

A few months earlier, I was in tears in the morning. Now I couldn't wait to get out of bed and nourish my soul!

I continued running and set a goal to run my first 5k. I began running three to five times per week and discovered that I always had incredible energy after my runs. I completed my first 5k right after my son, Nathan, was born!

Don and I had breakfast a few months later. He shared that the changes in me were obvious. Many people commented to him that I was changing. He shared that I was no longer selfish but becoming selfless. I was putting others' needs in front of my own and they were noticing it.

On June 2, 2008, I wrote in my journal:

> *"Good weekend. Been feeling pretty good for a long time."*

I changed my system and it changed the results in my life. I chose action over apathy. I chose not to be a victim and emerged victorious.

These lessons carried me through my daughter's struggles with addiction. They carried me through my wife's battle with cancer. They carried me through my time of being laid off from Microsoft. They carried me through my mother's sickness and eventual death. They carried me through my wife's second bout with cancer, and they are carrying me through my own bout with cancer.

On October 3, 2007, I was entering severe depression. I woke up with tears in my eyes. That was exactly 12 years ago. I'm writing this on October 3, 2019. My mood swings from bipolar are 100% gone. I have never experienced depression since. I have tons of energy and I'm living the life of my dreams. I'm on my 17th day of radiation treatment and I feel better than the day I started treatment. I feel the sun on my back, and I've decided that I'm going to bike 22 miles to radiation treatment again today.

The doctors tell me that the next four weeks are going to be very difficult. You might say I'm entering a season of drought. But I am not anxious. I trust in the Lord. He has carried me before and He will carry me during this season as well.

Thank You, Jesus, for the lessons You taught me in my pain 12 years ago. Thank You that You didn't remove my pain until I learned the lessons. Thank You that You helped me turn these lessons into habits, habits that carried me so many times and will carry me in the future. Thank You for the fruit from these lessons. Thank You for the vision that is becoming a reality, the vision of developing men. Thank You for the gift of writing. Thank You for replenishing my soul while I worship You on my bike rides in the sun listening to my favorite music.

And thank You for the cancer that was in my body a few months ago and will never return. If I hadn't had that cancer, I wouldn't have written this book. Jesus, I pray that my experiences will bring glory to You and positively influence those who I influence.

Amen

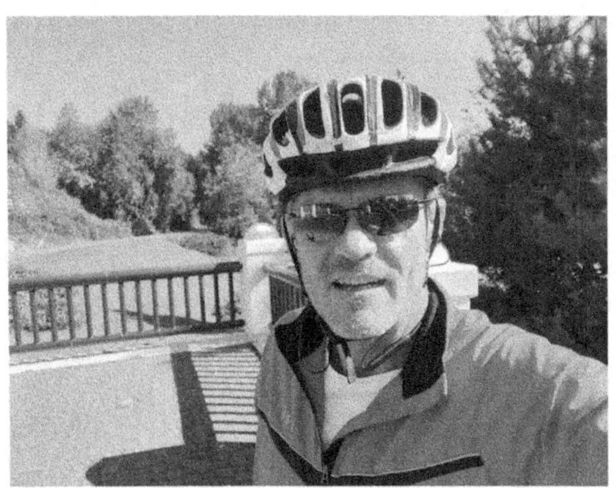

Questions to Consider

1. How does your outlook affect your attitude? Are there any shifts you need to make in your outlook to improve your attitude?

2. Have you ever experienced depression? How did you overcome it?

3. How can I help?

CHAPTER 13

10/21/2019

The Voice of Truth

"**D**ad, your neck is red. It's a deep dark red, about the color of the Washington Redskins' helmets!" Nathan said as we were snuggling watching the football game yesterday.

My neck is red. A physical representation of the molecular changes occurring in my flesh due to radiation. I've been at this for 40 days today. I'll have my 28th of 30 radiation treatments in a few hours.

The doctors and nurses have all promised a long list of side effects. Every time I visit them, they tell me "It's coming." Here are a few of the things they've promised:

- Sequelae of Xerostomia (Dry mouth)

- Dysphagia (Difficulty swallowing)

- Mucositis (Ulceration of the mouth)

- Weakness/fatigue

- Radiodermatitis (Redneck)

I've experienced a little bit of all of these symptoms. (I estimate I've lost about 40% of my saliva, I have some difficulty swallowing and occasional sores in my mouth, and I am definitely more tired. My neck is obviously very red as well.) But they don't list the three symptoms that have impacted me the most. My loss of taste, my emotional health, and my resultant weight loss.

I'd like to share a bit more of my journey in the following paragraphs as I believe I've learned some lessons that may help you.

Let's start with my weight. During my last visit, the nurse was very stern with me. "I'm concerned about your weight. It is the biggest determining factor for how quickly you'll recover."

"Why aren't you eating?" she asked.

"Food tastes awful. I just can't force it down," I responded.

"You're going to have to figure it out. If it was because of the pain, I'd give you pain medicine to help. I can't help you decide to eat even if you don't want to."

"I know, I know," I responded.

A month earlier my weight was 216 pounds, higher than it has been in more than 10 years. Today, it's 204 pounds, lower than it's been in six years. I'm losing about two pounds per week.

The nurse reminded me again that my full recovery would be fully dependent on my ability to maintain my weight.

I thanked her for her stern words and set a new goal to stabilize my weight.

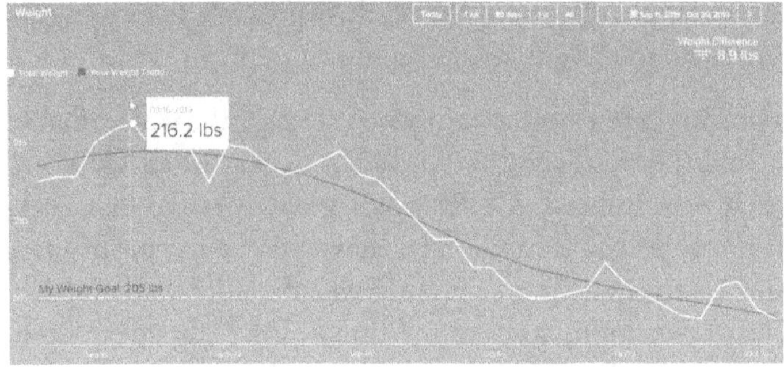

But my weight loss is a symptom of something much deeper. Something that a few bouts of uncontrollable sobbing and a conversation with a trusted advisor would have to reveal.

Our family loves the fall season. Football starts, the air is cool and crisp, the trees change colors, and it's simply beautiful in Washington state. Monica's birthday is at the end of September, and Debbie's birthday is only a few days later on the first of October.

As a family, we love to celebrate special occasions. Debbie always goes out of her way to cook everyone's favorite food and dessert. This year was no exception. This year she spent the morning prepping. Amanda came over. She'd made a pumpkin cheesecake and it looked delicious. She brought Monica special non-dairy ice cream.

A few weeks earlier, we all got together, and I barbecued the salmon Nathan and I caught. I seared the juices in over the hot barbecue. It was delicious. "Best salmon I've ever had," according to my father-in-law! I must admit, it was the best tasting salmon I'd ever had as well.

I fired up the barbecue and cooked a few slabs of the salmon Nathan and I caught a month earlier. As everyone gathered around the table, I couldn't get the words out as I was fighting tears, so I asked my father-in-law to pray instead.

I hesitantly put a piece on my plate fearing the worse, that it wouldn't taste as good as it did a few weeks earlier. My worst fears were realized. All flavor was gone. It tasted like cardboard and I could barely get it down. As I sat at the head of the table watching my family laugh and talk together, I felt an overwhelming knot in my throat. I quickly got up, put my plate in the sink, and rushed outside.

The tears began flowing uncontrollably. I went into my truck and shut the door so nobody would hear me. I sat in my truck and sobbed like a baby mourning the loss of my taste buds. The tears kept coming as I feared never being able to enjoy a good meal again. This fear came from deep inside, the same level of fear I'd felt when I was told I had cancer.

But then an all-too-familiar voice shocked me out of my tears.

"Seriously Damon? You're sobbing because you can't taste anything? What a baby. It's only taste. There are people who have lost a lot more than their taste. Grow up!"

That all-too-familiar voice of shame quickly put a stop to my tears. I went back into the house and tried to celebrate with my family. But try as I might, I simply couldn't snap myself out of it.

Visiting my mother-in-law didn't help. She'd fallen a few days earlier and couldn't move.

"Seriously, Damon? You've lost your taste and you're sobbing uncontrollably? Look at your mother-in-law. She's the one that should be sobbing; she can't move. Grow up!"

Truth is that my mother-in-law was in pretty serious condition. She ended up going to the emergency room that night because her pain was so extreme.

The next morning, I awoke and things didn't get any better for me. I cried as I said goodbye to my kids. I cried in my truck driving to work. I cried in my co-worker's office. I cried on the trip to radiation, and I cried with my head strapped down to the radiation table.

"Seriously, Damon? It's just your taste buds! Stop whining!"

Try as it might, that voice of shame didn't stop the tears.

I've surrounded myself with wise counselors. I have friends I can call at any time and they always listen and offer support. I knew I needed to talk to someone, and my immediate instinct was to call my counselor and close friend.

As I pulled into work, I got on the phone and called her.

"Hey. I was hoping you could help me identify the source of my tears," I choked out with tears flowing.

"Let's pray."

We prayed and she asked me what I heard during prayer.

"Well, it's not about food and it's not about taste. It's deeper than that."

"Where do you feel it?" she asked.

"In my belly," I responded. "I remember what you told me years ago. Emotional pain that I can feel in my belly is deep rooted."

"Enjoying a good meal together is one of my favorite things to do. As a family we draw close to one another when we are enjoying a good meal. Debbie and I draw close to each other over a good meal. Monica and I always celebrate over a good meal. Noelle and I have special meals together. We just love being together and enjoying a great meal," I said.

"And now I can't enjoy a great meal with the people I feel closest to," I sobbed.

"It's not about the food, Damon. It's about the connection you feel when you are enjoying food together," she said.

"And little Damon fears that the loss of food will result in a loss of connection to those you love the most."

"That's it!" I said.

"It's a lie, Damon. Don't listen to it. You'll have to learn new ways to connect with those you love the most. You can do it!"

"Pam, there's one more thing. I think you're right, but I think there's more," I said.

"We grew up poor. But at Christmas my mom took the money she'd saved all year long and cooked a feast that was fit for a king. These are my favorite memories as a family. We were closest during those times."

"You're right, Damon."

"But there's even more," I said.

"When I was a child and I came home from school, we were locked out. Mom didn't have anywhere to take us children, so we all lived in a park for a few days. Mom didn't have any food or shelter for us, so ultimately, we all had to go in different directions to different foster homes. I think I'm equating the loss of my taste buds with the loss of my family of origin as well. It's triggering the fear of abandonment I thought I'd worked through."

"You're right, Damon. But your family isn't going to abandon you. I want you to go home and hold that stuffed lion that I gave you," Pam said.

A few weeks earlier, Pam had a gift delivered to my home to give me courage as I went through radiation.

She bought me a stuffed lion, Aslan from *The Lion, the Witch, and the Wardrobe*. She told me this lion was symbolic because much like Lucy saw the lion and pursued him, so did I. She told me that the lion represented safety and security, and to hold him when little Damon was feeling scared. She reminded me that the lion represented Jesus, and Jesus would never leave me in the storm.

I thanked Pam for her wisdom and said goodbye. I went home and held that lion, Aslan. Those fears subsided and that voice of shame was squelched with the voice of truth.

The truth is my family loves me. We don't need food to be close to one another. That evening, I snuggled with Noelle on the couch. Nathan sat in my lap watching football a few days later. My wife hugged me and held me tightly as we prayed together. Monica wrote me a sweet note, invited me over to her new home, and we spent the evening together. Amanda encouraged me and told me how proud she was of me.

That voice of shame lost its oomph. I haven't mourned the loss of my taste buds since. In fact, miraculously, a few days later, I discovered some food that I can taste! Strawberry and blueberry Odwalla is delicious. Clam chowder is divine. Avocado toast is an incredible breakfast!

And Aslan, that lion that my wise counselor and friend gave me, was spending time bringing courage and strength where it was needed. I brought him to my mother-in-law as she was writhing in pain preparing for surgery.

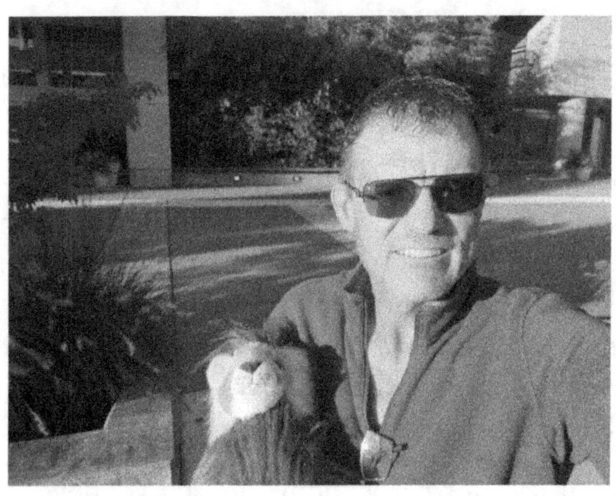

"That's Jesus," she said.

I watched the peace of God that transcends all understanding wash over her when I put Aslan on her pillow. He was watching over her while she was in surgery, and was on her pillow during her recovery. And he's with her right now in rehab as she prepares to come home.

That's Jesus.

Thank You, Jesus for watching over my mother-in-law as she recovers from surgery. Thank You for Pam and her wisdom in bringing that lion to me as a gift. Thank You for her wisdom in helping me hear the voice of truth and not the voice of shame. Thank You for my family and how they've each loved me in unique and special ways through this radiation journey. And thank You for the miracles that identified and now eradicated cancer from my body. Jesus, I pray that my words would inspire others who are unable to drown out the voice of shame and help them hear the voice of truth.

Amen

Questions to Consider

1. What are the voices in your head that are telling you lies? What is the voice of truth that you need to replace these voices with?

2. What are the rituals that pull your family closer together?

3. How can I help?

CHAPTER 14

10/25/2019

Finishing Strong

Jesus answered:
Love the Lord your God with all your heart, soul,
and mind. This is the first and most important
commandment. The second most important
commandment is like this one. And it is, "Love others
as much as you love yourself." All the Law of Moses
and the Books of the Prophets are based on these
two commandments.
— Matthew 22:37-40

Wahoo!

I'm done with cancer treatment!!

I'm cancer free!!!

Three days ago, I entered the UW Radiation Oncology department for my final treatment, day 41 of 41 for treatment 30 of 30. As I laid on the table for the final time with my family waiting in the lobby, I was filled with joy. The joy of knowing that I am now a cancer survivor. The joy that my body responded quite differently than most patients' bodies. (According to my radiologist, I'm an "anomaly" in terms of how well my body responded to radiation.)

Much like every day of radiation, I lay on the radiation table with my head strapped to the table with the mask. My favorite worship music played in the background and I gently moved my palms upward to praise Jesus for His hand on my life. The final song I heard during my final treatment was the same song I vowed to follow throughout my treatment.

Praise You in The Storm

And I'll praise You in this storm
And I will lift my hands
That You are who You are
No matter where I am
And every tear I've cried
You hold in Your hand
You never left my side
And though my heart is torn
I will praise You in this storm[vi]

I walked through the one-foot thick lead door and into the lobby to cheers! I banged the gong proclaiming, "I'm cancer free and I'm done!" I hugged the nurses and thanked them, and hugged my wife and older daughters, thanking them for being there to celebrate this accomplishment.

Unfortunately, my day didn't start as well as that moment. I live in Seattle and fall is upon us. It's been raining almost nonstop and the rivers are flooding from all the rain. It's no fun riding my bike in the rain, so it's been sitting in my garage.

The rain and going through cancer treatment have been a GREAT excuse to fall out of the routine that I've been doing three to six days per week for the last 12 years—cardio exercise for at least 30 minutes.

And I could feel it. My energy level was waning, and my positivity waned and became negativity. I spent more time on the phone and computer and less time with my family. And on this morning, the last morning of my treatment, I yelled at my wife. I argued with her and began blaming her for how I was feeling.

And then I broke down in tears.

"I'm sorry. I just need some freedom. I'm going to bike to UW for my final treatment."

"Honey, it's supposed to rain."

"I don't care. I need to go."

I reached for my headphones and couldn't find them. Turns out my truck had been broken into a few days earlier and in this moment, I discovered that they'd also gotten my headphones.

I came back in the house and asked my wife where her headphones were. I grabbed them, knowing that the headphones were part of the process for recharging.

"I love you. I'll see you soon," I said and jumped on my bike.

I pedaled up the long hill wheezing and thinking to myself, "You're crazy. You are on your final radiation treatment. You're supposed to be on your back on the couch from the pain and have a feeding tube to ensure that you have enough nourishment, and you're biking 15 miles?"

"Yup," I thought to myself. "I'm running on empty and I need to recharge."

So I kept pedaling. By the time I got to the trail, the sun started coming out. I stopped for a moment, put my headphones in, and turned on my worship playlist (a collection of Christian songs that speak to my soul and help me feel closer to God).

Minutes later, as I felt the sun beaming on my face and my favorite worship music playing in my ears, I looked up to see the beauty of God's creation. With my heart racing, I took my hands off the handlebars and raised them in worship while I sang words that have carried me through so many trials. The same words that carried me through this trial.

In Your Presence[vii]

As I stand here in Your presence
Of Your beauty I will always stand in awe
I reach my hands out to the heavens, yeah,
And I lift my voice to You alone.
To You alone

I remembered hearing this song while writing in my office, a few hours before my doctor's appointment to reveal the extent of my cancer. The tears flowed that day and I was overwhelmed with peace as I felt the presence of God flooding my soul letting me know that it was going to be ok.

The sun continued to shine, and I began pedaling harder, my heart pumping life-giving blood through my veins, eradicating the side effects of radiation, and eliminating any remaining cancer. I looked up and saw God's beauty through His creation. Lake Washington with Mt. Rainier in the distance.

And I felt alive. I was alive! Cancer tried to steal my life. It tried to steal my joy. When it failed, fear tried to take its place. If cancer wouldn't take my physical life, then certainly fear would take my spiritual and emotional life.

But fear failed as well. Try as it might, it failed. Fear did not steal my joy; in fact, I'd argue that fear led me to an even deeper joy. A joy that I couldn't have experienced if I hadn't fought the fear.

Every time I felt fear, I conquered it using the same tools that I learned years ago. I fought fear by making a decision. A decision for action, not apathy.

But not any action. My decision was always to take the action that would have the biggest impact at conquering my fear. I chose (and continue to choose) faith in the middle of fear, and that faith is what always eradicates fear.

Let me explain.

Debbie had just received the news that she had cancer for the second time. We were both gripped by fear. I tried to be strong for her, but I couldn't fake it anymore. I called my wise pastor, mentor, and friend Don.

With tears streaming down my face, I shared my fears. His response has changed my life and the lives of everyone I coach forever.

"Damon, fear is a spirit and you must conquer it the same way Jesus did. You must conquer spiritual battles with spiritual tools."

And he reminded me of the scripture that had helped me so many times in the past. The scripture I spoke out loud when I was gripped with depression. The scripture I spoke out loud on my morning walks when my daughter was stuck in addiction. The scripture that I spoke when I heard that I had cancer. The scripture that immediately eradicates my fear and replaces it with faith.

> *For God has not given me a spirit of fear, but of power and love and sound mind.*
> — 2 Tim 1:7

God gave me a spirit of power and love and sound mind.

As I continued pedaling, listening to worship music, and experiencing his majesty through nature, I experienced that power and love and sound mind. With His help, I found power to do what I didn't want to do, and experienced enormous peace (sound mind) in the process.

As I pulled into the hospital, the tears streamed from my eyes. "I'm a cancer survivor!" The next song captured my emotions.

All Creatures of Our God and King[viii]

All creatures of our God and King
Lift up your voice and with us sing
Oh, praise Him!
Alleluia!
Thou burning sun with golden beam
Thou silver moon with softer gleam
Oh, praise Him!
Oh, praise Him!
Alleluia!
Alleluia!
Alleluia!

The tears kept coming. I'd just beaten cancer.

"Alleluia" literally means to worship and rejoice. How could I not praise him? How could I not worship and rejoice? Alleluia, Alleluia, Alleluia, Alleluia, Alleluia, Alleluia!

I'm singing now. Alleluia, alleluia, alleluia!

Since this was my last radiation appointment, I met with my physician. Unfortunately, my primary radiologist was out, so I met with his resident who had never seen me.

He entered the room and introduced himself. "I'll be the resident seeing you through your treatment."

"That's great," I said, "but this is my last treatment."

The look on his face was priceless.

"Wow, you look incredible," he said.

"Thanks, I feel incredible. I just biked 15 miles to celebrate."

His jaw hit the floor. "That's unheard of. You biked 15 miles on your last day of treatment? Most people are barely able to make it in because they are in pain, out of energy, and taking nourishment from a feeding tube."

"Are you taking medicine to help you eat?" he asked.

"Nope. I haven't taken any medicine for pain during the whole treatment. Very little pain, only when swallowing occasionally," I responded.

"I'm blown away. Whatever you are doing, keep doing. It's working. Congratulations!" He shook my hand and walked out.

Whatever you're doing, keep doing. It's working.

I haven't done the research to support my theory, and I realize that everyone responds differently. That being said, I firmly believe that my body and my spirit have responded so well to treatment because I have chosen to obey the greatest commandments.

Jesus answered:
Love the Lord your God with all your heart, soul,
and mind. This is the first and most important
commandment. The second most important
commandment is like this one. And it is, "Love others
as much as you love yourself." All the Law of Moses
and the Books of the Prophets are based on these
two commandments.
— Matthew 22:37-40

By now it should be pretty obvious that I'm Christian and I've chosen to love God with all my heart, soul, and mind. That's obvious.

But I'm betting my obedience to the second part of this commandment isn't quite as obvious.

Love others as much as you love yourself. I could write an entire book on this one verse, but I want to try to summarize it here in hopes that I can give you the same paradigm shift that I had years ago that unquestionably is the single biggest factor (outside of my faith) in who I am today.

Love others as much as you love yourself.

I'd heard the verse a thousand times, and I bet you have too. But there is a subtle nuance that when you understand it and apply it, everything changes.

So, is it more important to love others or love yourself?

Before answering, I want you to think about this…

How much can you love others?

Simple.

As much as you love yourself.

So, if I want to love others MORE, how do I do it?

Simple.

Love yourself more.

Now what do you think? Is it more important to love others or to love yourself?

I want to argue that it is more important to love yourself because the more you love yourself, the more you can love others!

My argument this morning with my wife is proof of that. I hadn't been loving myself in the ways I knew I needed to and as a result, we got into an argument. The argument was about me EXPECTING HER to love me "more" because I had cancer and needed more love!

Do you see that? When I allowed myself the excuse of "I have cancer, so I don't have the energy to love myself," I started to decline rapidly. My decline resulted in my "needing love" versus "giving love," and we argued.

Fortunately, I knew what was going on. I was not loving myself and I needed to love myself by taking care of myself, regardless of the excuses in my mind. I needed to go for a bike ride in nature, listening to worship music with the sun shining on me. I needed to love myself so that I could love my wife and others around me.

So, I made the selfish decision to bike to my last treatment. Sorry for the sarcasm, but I know many of you don't love yourself because you feel like it is selfish. There's nothing farther from the truth. Loving yourself is the most selfless thing you can do because you can only love others as much as you love yourself.

And if that isn't enough justification for you, consider this. Jesus himself, the creator of the universe, said it was one of the two greatest commandments.

Love yourself.

This simple decision changed my life, broke the generational curses in my family, and is impacting thousands of people through my writing and coaching.

When I made this discovery years ago, I had no idea that it would also help me not only survive cancer but thrive from cancer.

One of the most important ways that I love myself is through exercise. I exercised for a minimum of 30 minutes of cardiovascular workouts, three to six times per week, every week for the last 12 years until I got cancer and couldn't do so.

Biking is obviously my favorite way of loving myself because biking allows me to increase my heart rate, enjoy God's creation, listen to worship music, and save me time in my commute.

So, I decided to celebrate my last day of radiation treatment by loving myself and biking 15 miles doing the same.

I firmly believe that the cumulative effect of loving God with all my heart, soul, mind, AND loving others as much as I love myself is why the impact of radiation is "an anomaly," according to my radiation oncologist, something that "I've almost never seen," according to my physical therapist. It's why I had the energy to bike 15 miles the last day, which is "unheard of" according to the resident radiation oncologist. I believe it's why I have almost no pain, and it's why I didn't need a feeding tube. I believe it's why my cancer was discovered, and I believe it's why I will be free of cancer for eternity.

I believe it's why I was able to write this book, and I believe it's why so many people are inspired by my story.

A little more than 20 years ago, I was in extreme pain. Separated from my wife and moving away from my baby daughter was the most painful thing I'd ever done. But as I wrote about in my first book, *Pain Drives Change*, that pain drove me to make the changes I needed to make to love myself and break the generational curses in my family. I chose action over apathy back then, and I continue to do so most every day of my life by following these two greatest commandments of loving God and loving others as much as I love myself!

And now I'm cancer free!

WAHOO!!!!!

Thank You, Jesus, that You showed me so many years ago how to love You and how to love myself. Thank You that I chose action and this action has rid my body of cancer. Thank You for showing me that loving myself is not "selfish" but "selfless" and thank You that because of this, my fears of radiation were not realized, but instead I'm an "anomaly." Thank You for the trial of cancer which has deepened my faith and given me the opportunity to share it with others through this story. Thank You in advance for the hope and inspiration this story will bring to so many who need it.

Amen

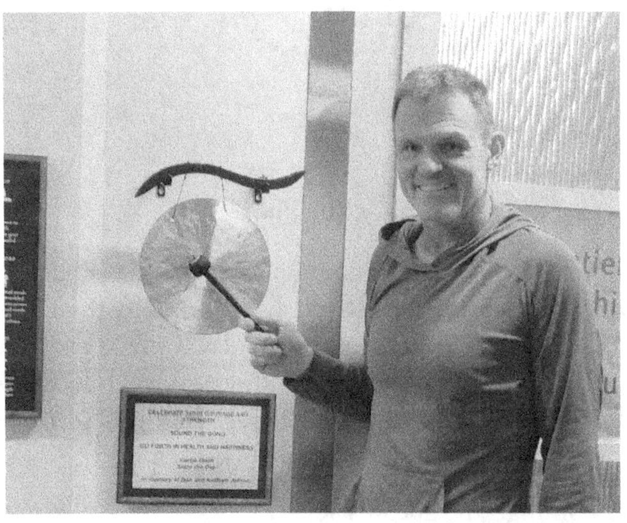

Questions to Consider

1. Is loving your neighbor as much as you love yourself selfish or selfless?

2. How do you love yourself so that you can love others more?

3. Are you loving yourself enough during this season? What needs to change?

4. How can I help?

CHAPTER 15

Decision Time: Apathy or Action?

Action Plan

Six months ago, I felt a lump on my neck. I was busy and made every excuse possible to avoid going to the doctor. I still remember it like it was yesterday. I met a friend for lunch. I was close to the doctor's office and so I decided to call and see if they had time that day. They did, so instead of going back to work, I went to the doctor.

"It's nothing," the doctor said.

I could have easily listened to him and gone back to work. Fortunately for me, my wife had cancer two times before, my sister had cancer, and my mom had cancer. Their misfortune with having cancer inspired me to action.

"I'm worried about it," I said.

"I'm not, but take some vitamin C and call me in a week," he said.

"I'd like to come back in a week instead," I said.

"OK. We'll see you in a week."

I immediately scheduled the appointment for the next week. This small decision to take immediate action made a very big impact.

A week later, nothing had changed.

"I'm still not worried," the doctor said.

"I am," I retorted.

In lieu of remaining apathetic about my lump, I chose action.

"I want to know what it is," I said.

"OK. We'll schedule a CT Scan, but I'm doing it for you," the doctor responded.

A week later, the scan was inconclusive. My doctor called me, knowing I wouldn't accept this as an answer.

"I'm referring you to a specialist," he said.

A week later, the specialist said the same thing.

"I'm not worried about it."

Once again, I didn't accept this answer.

"I am. My sister had cancer, my wife had it twice, and so did my mom. I want to know for sure," I said.

"OK. We'll do a needle biopsy under ultrasound to be certain," she said.

A week later, on May 28, 2019, I got the call. I was at work and walked into a spare conference room.

"You have cancer," she said.

I choked back the tears.

"How serious?"

"Not sure, but it is very treatable."

Over the next five months, my family and I went on a roller-coaster ride with our emotions. Each step of the way I was faced with a simple decision:

Apathy or Action

And every time, I chose action. I'm alive, healthy, and cancer free today because of that small choice to take action.

Where would I be if I'd chosen apathy? Maybe I'd be dead.

But I'm not. I'm alive and stronger than I was before.

That's how it works. Apathy paralyzes, but action energizes. But when we are stuck in fear, many times apathy takes over and we become victims instead of emerging victorious.

Over time, this attitude of apathy will destroy us and everyone around us.

But the decision to take action will change everything, and it will impact everyone around you for the better.

I'd like to share one last story of when I learned how the power of action to conquer fear resulted in one of the best experiences of my life.

People who know me say I'm one of the most passionate, positive, and energizing people they've ever met. But I haven't always been that way. I've struggled with being lazy and listless my whole life.

But I've always had a dream of completing a triathlon. Unfortunately, my fear of not having enough energy to complete it made me apathetic toward the idea of ever doing it. This resulted in even less energy and motivation to try.

One day I chose action. I decided I was going to do a triathlon the following summer. I couldn't swim, I didn't have a bike, and I hated running.

But I bought a bike right before going on vacation and I brought it with me. As a side note, I bought the bike because my best friend began biking to work a year earlier, and he loved it, which inspired me to get my own bike. Choose your friends wisely because you will become the average of the five people you are closest to.

My friend and I went for my first bike ride on that vacation. I loved it. The next day he jumped on his bike and rode up a hill that no human in their right mind should bike up. And the next day, he did it again, and the next day, again. I promised myself that I'd ride up that hill the following year. Jokingly, I looked at the lake and said, "One day, I'll swim across this lake," knowing that I couldn't swim a single stroke!

I began biking to work and I loved it. But I avoided the decision to sign up for a triathlon, even though I'd committed to myself that I was going to do it.

Weeks passed and I felt more and more internal pressure to sign up even though I couldn't swim.

Once again, I had a decision to make. Remain apathetic and avoid pursuing my dream or take action and sign up.

I signed up.

Small choice. Big impact!

That decision triggered another decision to get swimming lessons. After a few lessons, I was able to swim (if you can call it that). Twenty-five yards in the pool and I was out of breath. But I kept going, knowing I had to swim 400 yards in a few months.

On July 21, 2013, I completed my first triathlon and successfully swam (with a lot of back floating) 400 yards!

I was hooked, so I immediately signed up for the next year and next level.

This time the swim was 800 yards, twice as far.

Once again, I put off the start of training because I was afraid I wouldn't be able to swim the 800 yards. I chose apathy instead of action and it was paralyzing me.

Finally, I made the small decision and in May of 2014, I started training. My bike rides were incredible, but my swims were atrocious.

I kept training. But things never improved. I was still out of breath at 25 yards. I didn't quit. I kept training and I kept asking people that could swim how they did it.

One day, I was swimming and after 400 yards, I decided to try a slightly different breathing technique.

WAHOO! I'm swimming and I'm not out of breath—500 yards, 600 yards, 800 yards! WAHOO!

I decided to set a goal to swim a mile. The next week, I swam 1000 yards. A few days later 1200 yards. And a few days after that, a mile! I could swim a mile where a few weeks earlier, I couldn't swim 25 yards! And I loved it!

I was in peak condition and I was ready for this triathlon. I went for a swim a few weeks before in the lake, and for some unknown reason, I could barely swim a few strokes before getting winded!

I was gripped with fear. What was I going to do? The triathlon was only a few weeks away and 800 yards is a long swim. What would happen if I couldn't finish the swim? Maybe I should cancel my registration just in case.

I wrestled in fear for a few days. I was paralyzed and impossible to be around. I'm not a quitter, so quitting simply wasn't option. I remembered a lesson I'd learned when my daughter was only a toddler. A lesson about the importance of pushing through fear. A lesson that I've applied to my own life and the way I raise my children and coach my clients.

In the book *If You Want to Walk on Water You've Got to Get Out of the Boat*[ix], John Ortberg talks about where we build or lose self-esteem. As much as it seems like self-esteem would be built by being encouraged or words like "you're doing a great job," it isn't. Self-esteem is built when you are facing fear and you choose action. In choosing action and pushing through our fears, we build our self-esteem.

He shares the example of a child standing on the edge of the pool, afraid to jump in. If the child doesn't push through and jump into the pool, his or her self-esteem plummets. However, if the child pushes through and jumps into the pool, his or her self-esteem grows.

Furthermore, the role of a father is critical here. The father standing in the pool, encouraging the child to jump and, more importantly, providing the safety, is just enough for the child to conquer their fear and jump.

"I did it, daddy. I did it!" the child proclaims after jumping. Their self-esteem grows and they are ready to do it again, maybe even jump farther or in the deep end!

Alternately, "I can't," the child proclaims and walks away. Self-esteem plummets and the next time they have a fear, they won't conquer it and it will plummet even more.

Here I was. Faced with the same fear the child has before jumping into the pool. Paralyzed about the "what-ifs."

After about two days I decided. "I'm going to do it." I got up early the next day and went to my favorite swimming spot. I watched the sunrise as I put on my wetsuit, gripped with fear that I still wouldn't be able to swim more than 10 strokes. But I pushed through. The warm water on my face and hands energized me. I started swimming.

1...2...3...4...5...6...7...8...9...10 strokes. "Wahoo, I'm not breathing hard!" I thought to myself. So, I kept swimming and swimming and swimming. I swam a mile that day and barely lost my breath!

A few weeks later, I completed the longest triathlon I've ever done, beating my best time for the swim and enjoying it more than almost anything I've ever done! I was elated, and my self-esteem took a major boost. I felt like I could conquer the world.

A few weeks later, I brought my wetsuit to Keller Ferry, determined to swim across the lake like I'd jokingly said I'd do a few years earlier when I couldn't swim a stroke. It was one of the most incredible experiences of my life. The water was calm and warm. The sun was shining. I swam all the way across the lake! I'll never forget the joy I experienced.

I was so elated that I decided I was going to bike that hill the next day, the hill that a few years earlier I never thought doable. So, I did. I biked the entire hill!

I was so elated, that I decided to sign up for a 100-mile bike ride (the most I'd ever done was 30 miles). So, I did. It, too, was one of the most incredible experiences of my life!

The next year, I trained and performed my longest triathlon ever. The swim of nearly a mile was more enjoyable than almost any I'd experienced.

I was so elated that I decided to swim across the lake and back a few years later at the same place I'd swam across the year before! And I did! 2.4 miles!

I was so elated by my new found athleticism that I biked the same hill—on five different days! One day I biked the hill and felt so great that I biked another 20 miles through the backroads with beautiful wheat fields to visit my mom's gravesite, and I felt so great after that I biked the 25 miles to get back to the camp spot!

Looking back, those simple decisions to take action when faced with fear resulted in some of the most incredible experiences of my life. Experiences that I would never have enjoyed had I chosen apathy in the face of fear.

Where would I be today if I hadn't taken action when faced with the fear of swimming? I can't say, but I bet I would be overweight and depressed. I bet my relationship with my family wouldn't be as strong. I bet that cancer treatment would have taken a much more severe toll on my body (and maybe even taken my life).

I bet I wouldn't be writing this book that you are reading now and challenging you to take action in your fear.

I don't know what your fear is. Perhaps it's cancer, perhaps you're having money problems, perhaps you are afraid to change jobs or afraid to discipline your children. Perhaps you're afraid to confront your spouse about issues that are tearing your marriage apart. I don't know. Perhaps you're afraid to see the doctor for fear of the prognosis. Perhaps you're afraid to start exercising or afraid to let others read your writing.

I don't know what you're afraid of. It doesn't matter.

You have a choice. Will you choose apathy or will you choose action? It's a small choice but it will have a big impact.

I'm here to encourage you and challenge you along the way. I know you can do it.

Thank You, Jesus, for the opportunity to write this book. Thank You that I've fought cancer and won. Thank You that You inspired me to write this book for others to benefit. Thank You for my sister who has beaten cancer twice. Thank You for my wife who walked the path before me and beat cancer twice. Thank You for my mom who beat cancer. Thank You for my friend Ted and his courage as he fights cancer and the courage he gave me as I fought cancer. Thank You for the men who gathered around me multiple times to pray. Thank You for the doctors and their wisdom and thank You for Your divine guidance in finding and eliminating the cancer from my body. Thank You for the long life that my family will enjoy because my wife and I are cancer free. And thank You for the encouragement this story will offer so many people who are in need of some encouragement.

Amen

> All praise goes to God, Father of our Lord Jesus, the Anointed One. He is the Father of compassion, the God of all comfort. He consoles us as we endure the pain and hardship of life so that we may draw from His comfort and share it with others in their own struggles.
> — 2 Corinthians 1:3-4

P.S. I'll end this with what I like to call the four magic words.

How can I help?

If you'd like some encouragement I'd love to help. Please schedule a free call with me and let's conquer your fears together. www.changeYOUniversity.org/action

Damon Stoddard

12/10/2019

The Story Isn't Over....

*So, if you think you are standing firm, be careful that
you don't fall!*
— 1 Corinthians 10:12

Will you allow me the freedom to be 100% transparent? I postponed the publication of this book because the story isn't over. I thought it was over. I thought I'd finished my cancer treatment and I would quickly return to life as normal.

I boasted about how I didn't experience most of the negative side effects of radiation treatment that the experts said I would. I boasted about how I had a ton of energy. People saw me and told me how I was one of the most positive and energy filled people they'd ever met.

"Inspiring" was the word that almost everyone who read my blogs or interacted with me used.

Truth be told, I felt fantastic. I'd beaten cancer, written a book, and inspired a lot of people in the process. Cancer was gone, my body needed a rest and my emotions needed a rest.

That was just the excuse I needed to become apathetic and stop doing the very things that I boasted about a few weeks earlier.

> *So, if you think you are standing firm, be careful that you don't fall!*
> — 1 Corinthians 10:12

I was standing firm. I had no idea I was about to fall.

Recall I've talked extensively about one of my favorite sayings from Dr. Deming:

Your system is perfectly designed to get you the results you are getting

Dr. Deming offered his services to the American automobile industry in the late 40's following World War II. They declined. Japan, however, was rebuilding and invited him to teach their management and engineers about quality.

One story talks about a manufacturing company that hired Deming to help them with quality. They were struggling to produce quality products and continually blamed their people for the issues. They hired Deming. After touring the manufacturing plant and observation, Deming produced his final report to management. His recommendations and results were not what management expected.

He shared that the *people were not the source of the problem.* Instead, he pointed out issues in the manufacturing processes and the management practices within the firm.

Improving quality would require improving these systems. Management heeded his words and began a relentless pursuit of continuous improvement in their systems. As a result, quality improved without changing the people.

Japan made Deming into a hero, and in 1951, created the Deming prize for companies that were leaders in applying his techniques to improve quality.

Deming repeatedly pointed to the *system* as the source of the majority of the issues he encountered. Near his time of death, Deming reflected on the thousands of problems he'd encountered and solved. He reported that 96% of these problems were because of issues with the underlying system. 96%! Furthermore, he pointed out that improvement of these systems was the responsibility of management.

Your system is perfectly designed to get you the results you are getting

I took this quote to heart, and in 2009, I began viewing my life from a systems' perspective. For example, I looked at our spending and implemented a few simple systems to get it under control. (I sent Debbie a paycheck every payday and we adjusted our spending based on a cash system).

I looked at our relationship and realized that even though I said it was important, my "system" didn't support this statement. Time together was the "critical factor" in improving our relationship, yet time together was the LAST item on my calendar. We made a simple change and began prioritizing date nights, weekends away, and regular "business meetings." Our system changed and our results changed too. We were closer than we'd ever been.

We implemented "systems" in many other areas of our lives—family relationships, friendships, ministry, etc. As a result, we saw incredible growth in all areas of or lives.

I applied systems' thinking to help resolve many of the problems I'd experienced my entire life, the biggest one being my battle with bipolar. As a result, my mood swings virtually disappeared. My entire life I'd struggle with the highs and lows of bipolar. Unfortunately, nothing I did made a significant impact. It wasn't until I applied systems' thinking to the problem that I finally got it under control and kept it under control.

I shared my journey out of depression earlier in this book, but I didn't share the impact of the other side of bipolar-mania or hypomania. To be honest with you, I'd pretty much forgotten about this side of bipolar.

My system worked so well at stabilizing my moods that when I told people I was bipolar, they stared at me in disbelief.

Honestly, I didn't think much of it when cancer struck and I had to take time off from regular exercise, eating regularly, and consistently sleeping.

I felt so great through the cancer and incredibly elated from my occasional bike rides that I began forgetting about the importance of my system at maintaining my moods.

When cancer was over, I gave myself the excuse to take some time off of exercising regularly so my body could rebuild. I gave myself the excuse of sleeping irregularly instead of the consistency I'd done over the previous 10 years. I gave myself the excuse of eating more inconsistently (after all, food didn't taste good!). I gave myself the excuse of skipping my morning habits of time alone in the Bible, in prayer, being thankful, and encouraging others. I gave myself the excuse of not praying regularly with Debbie. I gave myself the excuse of not taking my anti-depressant regularly, and I got so busy that I stopped going to church regularly.

Before I knew it, the worst part of me started to take over. I stopped prioritizing time with Debbie (after all, food didn't taste good so spending time together over good food didn't make sense!). I stopped prioritizing time with my kids. I started snapping at everyone I loved when they tried to have a conversation with me. Debbie and I began arguing regularly. I criticized my kids for their attitudes when my own attitude was the problem.

My hands started falling asleep while sleeping, and I began waking up very early in the morning, unable to go back to sleep. My mind started racing, and I began setting enormous goals that could never be achieved.

And I continued to not exercise.

My system that had worked flawlessly for nearly a dozen years was spinning out of control and I didn't even realize it.

Pain drives change.

One day, my wife and I got into an argument. I was too busy focusing on what mattered to me to listen to her, so I kept doing my own thing. She was furious (rightfully so). She drove away, leaving me wondering what I'd done. A few days later, we had a conversation that finally shocked me into reality.

She asked me if I was manic and insisted that I start taking my medication. Unfortunately, I didn't have my medication available and it was a few more days before I could start taking it again.

Those next few days were very difficult for me. In a little over a month, I'd began destroying the most precious relationships in my life. I'd stopped taking care of myself at a time when my body and emotions needed it the most, right after completing cancer treatment.

It was only a matter of time before my elevated moods caused irreparable damage. Something needed to change, and it needed to change quickly.

I quickly confessed my struggles with a few men that I meet with regularly, and I asked for their help and accountability. I called my friend and counselor, and she recommended I give Debbie decision authority over when I could taper off of the medication I use to stabilize my moods.

Years ago, another wise counselor, Dr. Jim Talley, taught me a few things that have radically transformed my life. He shared this:

> *Integrity is the time span between mess-up and*
> *fess-up.*
> — Dr. Jim Talley

I realized I'd messed up with my wife by treating her so poorly in my manic state. I sat down with her, held her hand and asked forgiveness. She quickly forgave me.

I realized I messed up with my 13-year-old daughter, Noelle. We went to coffee. I gave her my phone and told her I didn't want to spend time on it, I wanted to spend time with her and that it was getting in the way. I asked her forgiveness and for the first time I shared that I had bipolar, but that I'd be ok. She quickly forgave me. A few days later, she wrote me the most heartfelt note I've ever received from her.

I realized I messed up with my 11-year-old son, Nathan. I asked him to breakfast, gave him my phone, and told him I didn't want to spend time on my phone. Instead, I wanted to focus my time on him. I shared that I have bipolar, but that I'd be ok. And we proceeded to have the best conversation of our lives for more than an hour.

Dr. Talley taught me another thing as well. It's simple, profound, and the best systems' thinking you can apply to any relationship in your life:

> *The quality of your relationships is determined by the amount of quality time you spend alone together.*
> — Dr. Jim Talley

In my hypomanic state, I stopped spending quality time with my wife and children. Unfortunately, one of the most significant side effects of bipolar that affects me is my ability to hyperfocus. This unique ability has resulted in a book written in 45 days, a thriving coaching business, competing in triathlons, a very successful career, and not only surviving cancer, but writing a book during it and inspiring others because of it.

Unfortunately, my hyperfocus becomes a tractor beam. The tractor beam that we see on sci-fi movies. It grabs your ship and it pulls you into the enemy's ship. Nothing can be done to escape the tractor beam. It just keeps pulling you in and before you know it, you are a prisoner on the enemy's ship. This is how it is with me. The tractor beam of hyperfocus grabs me, and I cannot escape it. It pulls me away from my family and loved ones. It pulls me away from relationships.

It pulls me away from taking care of myself. And if I'm not careful, it wreaks havoc on my world.

Fortunately, my wife loved me enough to help me see the tractor beam had gotten me, and help me begin to escape it. And fortunately, Dr. Talley gave me the antidote to help improve our relationship. Quality time. The same quality time that we had "systematized" and worked extremely well before I was struck with cancer.

We are praying together regularly again, a practice that statistics show reduces the divorce rate to less than one in 1000^x. We are spending quality time alone regularly, taking walks, and riding in the car (without my phone). We are having business meetings again and discussing our relationship, and I have my small group of men holding me accountable to getting back on track. We've re-instituted the system that has worked well for more than 15 years, and once again, it is producing results.

I'm sleeping more regularly now. I've discovered a simple trick that keeps my hands from falling asleep while I sleep and I'm getting enough sleep finally. I'm starting to eat more food more regularly as well.

What goes up must come down.

I'm no longer in the hypomanic state that I experienced the past few weeks. Unfortunately, I'm slipping into a mild depression.

As I feel myself slipping into this mild depression, I am faced with a choice. The same choice I faced throughout my journey with cancer. It's a small choice, but it will have a big impact.

I have to decide if I'm going to be a victim of bipolar. Will I allow the depression that I so boldly proclaimed was 100% gone a few chapters ago to envelope me? Apathy would say that bipolar is biological, I was born with it, and it is out of my control. Apathy would say I must accept the mood swings and prepare myself for the onslaught of depression.

But there's another choice. It's a very small choice, but when made it will have a big impact. That choice is action. Will I choose to be paralyzed with fear of depression, or will I choose the action that has proven itself over the past 12 years to stabilize my moods?

The answer is simple. I'm choosing action. The consequences of apathy are too great. I'm choosing action. I didn't feel like going for a run today. I haven't felt like exercising in more than a month and a half.

IT DOESN'T MATTER HOW I FEEL!!!

If I listened to my feelings, I'd be crying myself to sleep right now and I'd be able to justify this decision.

Last night, when I barely felt enough energy to have a conversation with my kids, I made the decision. I decided that I was going to start exercising again today. I decided that I was going to do it at least three times per week for at least 30 minutes with my heart rate elevated. I laid out my exercise clothes before I went to bed, much like I've done for the past 12 years. When I got up in the dark, I put them on. I wore them in the car as we took the kids to school, and I wore them while I had breakfast. Then I wore them in the truck as I drove to the trail. I put my new headphones on, turned on my favorite worship music, and I began running.

My legs felt like lead and my heart rate quickly elevated to the point of being uncomfortable. And the life-giving blood began flooding my body and my brain. The sun shined on my face for a few brief moments and my favorite worship songs played in my ears.

"This is REALLY hard," I thought to myself.

"But I'm alive!"

I'm alive!

I'm alive!

I beat cancer!

I am healthy enough to exercise, and I'll beat depression again!

Four miles later, I emerged drenched in sweat even though it was only 40 degrees out.

I rushed home and started writing, knowing that in my failures of the past month and a half, I might be able to inspire those who are struggling right now.

I don't know what you are going through. But I know this. You have a choice to make. It's a small choice but it will have a big impact.

Don't choose apathy. Choose action.

Thank You, Jesus for pain. Thank You for the changes that come when we have the courage to face our pain and choose action. Thank You for my wife who had the courage to invoke pain on me recently when I began wreaking havoc on those I love the most. Thank You that my family loves me. Thank You for the wisdom You've given me and the ability to inspire others through it. Thank You that I am bipolar, and the pain it invokes forces me to take care of myself so that I can love others more. Thank You for this book and the people who are reading it. I pray that my story would inspire them in their pain and as a result the changes would be transformative for them and all they love.

Amen

Endnotes

i. Hall, Mark and Herms, Bernie. (2006). Praise You in the Storm [Recorded by Casting Crowns]. On *Lifesong* [album]. Brentwood, TN: Reunion Records. (2005)

ii. Stoddard, Damon. (2016). *Pain Drives Change.*

iii. Camp, Jeremy. (2002) In Your Presence (Recorded by Jeremy Camp). On *Jeremy Camp Stay* (album). BEC Recordings.

iv. Bennett, H. (Producer), & Nimoy, L. (Director). (1986.) *Star Trek IV- The Voyage Home* [Motion picture]. United States: Paramount Pictures.

v. Kim, C.M. *Carcinoma of Unknown Primary: The Role of Transoral Robotic Surgery.* [PowerPoint slides]. Retrieved from https://1drv.ms/p/s!AsI3x0k-8Yv09bJz58-2pL_Qdt44ZQ.

vi. Hall, Mark and Herms, Bernie. (2006). Praise You in the Storm [Recorded by Casting Crowns]. On *Lifesong* [album]. Brentwood, TN: Reunion Records. (2005)

vii. Camp, Jeremy. (2002) In Your Presence (Recorded by Jeremy Camp). On *Jeremy Camp Stay* (album). BEC Recordings.

viii. Draper, William Henry. (1919) All Creatures of Our God and King, (Recorded by David Crowder Band). On *Can You Hear Us* (album). Sparrow Records.

ix. Ortberg, John. (2008). *If You Want to Walk on Water You've Got to Get Out of the Boat.* Zondervan Publishing.

x. Lawrence, Arlyn. (2012). *God Kids? Pray First, Open Mouth Second.* Retrieved from https://arlynjoylawrence.com/2012/01/.

Biography

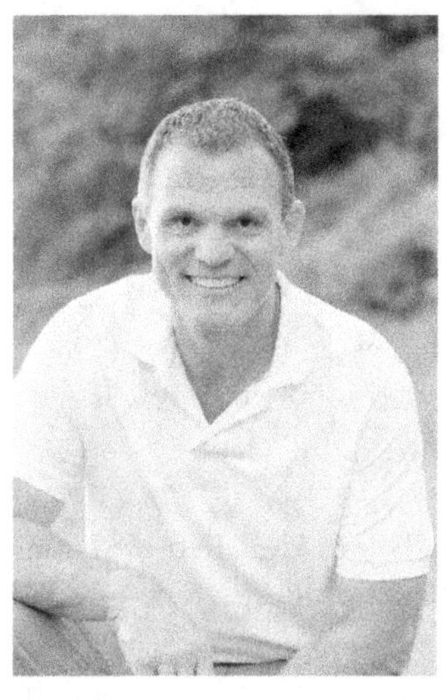

Damon Stoddard wrote his first book, *Pain Drives Change*, in 45 days. In this highly acclaimed book, Damon shares his personal transformation of overcoming divorce and building the family of his dreams. This book became the foundation for Change YOUniversity where he coaches men to build the families of their dreams and break the generational curses in their families forever.

In Damon's second book, *Apathy or Action*, Damon shares his personal journey of fighting cancer that has inspired countless people to take action when facing fear in their own lives

With over 25 years of professional experience as a change leader at Microsoft and Honeywell, Damon has a proven history of driving systematic, transformational change in organizations and individuals and has won numerous awards for his work. Damon has successfully applied these same principles to build a thriving men's ministry and small groups ministry in his church. Today, he is the Vice President of Discipleship for one of the premier Christian junior football programs in the nation where he mentors over 60 football coaches and more than 100 young men each year to put God first in their lives.

Together, he and his wife, Debbie, live near Seattle and enjoy the family of their dreams together.

You can find more information at:

www.changeYOUNiversity.org

Change YOUniversity

Reader,

If you've reached this point you've likely read my entire book. I'm praying that my story inspired you to take action in the areas of your life that are causing you the greatest pain. Remember, pain drives change, and pain is a gift from God. When it is more painful to stay the same than it is to change, change happens automatically.

If you are struggling to take action, or don't know what the best next steps are, I'd love to help. Change YOUniversity is a coaching system that has and is transforming people's lives, and I'm certain it can help you as well.

I'm offering a free call for the readers of my book to help you take action and make the changes you want to make.

It's a small choice, but I promise you it will have a big impact on your life.

Schedule your free call by going to the link below:

www.changeyouniversity.org/action

Damon

www.ingramcontent.com/pod-product-compliance
Lightning Source LLC
Chambersburg PA
CBHW061801250726
48657CB00001B/230